Gastrointestinal Health

Also by Steven R. Peikin, M.D.
The Feel Full Diet

Gastrointestinal Health

*A Self-Help Nutritional Program to
Prevent, Cure, or Alleviate Irritable Bowel
Syndrome, Ulcers, Heartburn, Gas, Constipation,
and Many Other Digestive Disorders*

Steven R. Peikin, M.D.

Recipes by Cheryl Clifford Marco, R.D.

HarperPerennial
A Division of HarperCollinsPublishers

A hardcover edition of this book was published in 1991 by HarperCollins Publishers.

HarperCollins books may be purchased for educational, business, or sales promotional use. For information, please call or write: Special Markets Department, HarperCollins Publishers, Inc., 10 East 53rd Street, New York, NY 10022. Telephone: (212) 207-7528; Fax: (212) 207-7222.

First HarperPerennial edition published 1992.

Designed by Joan Greenfield

The Library of Congress has catalogued the hardcover edition as follows:

Peikin, Steven R.
    Gastrointestinal health: a self-help nutritional program to prevent, cure, or alleviate irritable bowel syndrome, ulcers, heartburn, gas, constipation, and many other digestive disorders/by Steven Peikin.—1st ed.
        p. cm.
    Includes index.
    ISBN 0-06-016497-2
    1. Gastrointestinal system—Diseases—Popular works.   I. Title.
RC806.P45   1991
616.3 30654—dc20   90-55547

ISBN 0-06-098405-8 (pbk.)

94 95 96 DT/HC 10 9 8

To Lori, with love

Contents

Acknowledgments

I would like to thank the dietitians at Thomas Jefferson University Hospital, the United Weight Control Corporation, and the Jefferson Nutrition Support Team for their excellent nutritional care of my patients and also their help with this book; the medical students, fellows in gastroenterology, and other colleagues at Jefferson Medical College who aided in the development of *Gastrointestinal Health;* Susan Gordon, M.D., Larry Friedman, M.D., and Larry Miller, M.D., for their thoughtful comments and review of the manuscript; Laura Hill, R.D., and Barbara Whedon, R.D., for their assistance in recipe writing; Liz Emory, R.D., for assistance in preparation of the manuscript; Joyce Scott for technical assistance in the preparation of the manuscript; and Robert S. Dubin for his wise counsel.

For their help in developing specific chapters of *Gastrointestinal Health*, my special thanks to former fellow in gastroenterology David Stampfl, M.D.; Vicki Schwartz, M.S., R.D.; Brenda Byrne, M.D., of the Department of Psychiatry; and Patricia Vogel, B.A., former nutritional lecturer to Weight Watchers, United Kingdom.

I'd like to thank David Rorvik of Proteus, Inc., for his help in book concept development; Tom Miller, my editor, who improved the manuscript enormously; and Nancy Baggett, noted recipe writer and author of several cookbooks, for her help in recipe development.

I wish to express a special debt of gratitude to Josleen Wilson, author of *Woman, Your Body, Your Health,* and many other health books, for her valuable help in the preparation of the manuscript. And, finally, my thanks to Cheryl Clifford Marco, R.D., Manager of Outpatient Nutrition, Thomas Jefferson University Hospital, and author of the recipe section of *Gastrointestinal Health,* for her assistance in the preparation and review of all the other sections of the book.

This book is intended to help people better understand gastrointestinal symptoms and disorders. It should not be used as a means of self-diagnosis, since symptoms of relatively innocuous disorders are often confused with those of more serious diseases. A definitive diagnosis should always be made by a qualified physician.

As with all new dietary regimens, the Self-Help Nutritional Program should only be used in the context of a broader course of treatment as determined by a physician. The reader is advised that this dietary approach may not be appropriate in treating certain symptoms and disorders. In particular, this program is not recommended for people with acute pancreatitis, acute cholecystitis, intestinal obstruction, diverticulitis, or moderately or very active stages of Crohn's disease and ulcerative colitis.

Introduction

*Y*ou have a problem that's driving you crazy. Stomach pain, cramps or spasms, queasiness, frequent constipation or intermittent diarrhea, heartburn—all are signs that something is out of whack with your digestive system. Maybe you've been told you have irritable bowel syndrome (IBS) or "colitis," a catch-all term used to describe bouts of severe spasm followed by diarrhea or constipation or both. Perhaps when you're under stress you suddenly double over with stomach cramps and have to race to the bathroom. You might wake up in the mornings with what a patient of mine calls a "grungy" stomach. Or maybe in the middle of the night you feel acid rise in your throat, waking you out of a sound sleep.

Or maybe, like many people who come to me at the Jefferson Digestive Disease Service in Philadelphia, you have been diagnosed with more than one GI problem—perhaps a duodenal ulcer *and* a poorly functioning gallbladder. Your family doctor has told you to use milk products for your ulcer, but they aggravate your gallbladder pain. GI disturbances often trigger each other, and perhaps the most frustrating part of solving these problems is that what's soothing for one set of symptoms seems to aggravate another.

Virtually everyone, even people with cast-iron stomachs, suffers a bout of gastrointestinal distress from time to time as a reaction to stressful living, erratic diet, or temporary illness. Generally, as the event that triggered the symptom passes, so does the symptom. For many people, however, digestive problems are long-standing, provoked by almost anything, and often unrelieved, or only partly relieved, by medication.

More than 80 million Americans live with and suffer from chronic digestive problems. These sufferers may be of any age and background —for GI problems cross all barriers of age and economics—but a surprising number are between twenty-five and forty-five years of age. More than 60 percent are women. Next to the common cold, digestive ailments account for more absences from work and more visits to the doctor than any other condition. Symptoms may be continuous, with daily pain or discomfort, or they may subside for days or weeks at a time, only to come back again, without seeming provocation. Symptoms may be always mild or always severe, or they may swing from bad to worse.

GI symptoms are impossible to ignore, often revolving around meals, business lunches, and social occasions. The pleasure/pain syndrome becomes integrated into daily life: you enjoy eating something, then suffer the consequences. Chronic GI symptoms don't just go away. In fact, many tend to worsen with age: the longer you have them, the more aggravating they become.

Most treatments for GI problems involve medication. Year after year, GI drugs top the pharmaceutical best-seller lists. The cost to Americans of ulcer disease alone is $3.2 billion annually. Ranitidine (Zantac) alone sold worldwide well in excess of $1 billion last year, gaining it a place in the *Guinness Book of World Records*. We spend almost half a billion dollars a year on laxatives.

Yet, overall, drug therapy for GI problems has been notoriously unreliable. The most common and troublesome conditions, such as IBS, respond poorly to drugs of any kind. Although some GI drugs seem to correct problems virtually overnight, many are only partly effective and laden with potentially serious side effects. And at best, relief with drugs is only temporary, so taking the medication becomes a steady routine.

The Link Between Nutrition and Disease

It has taken science a long time to make the connection between diet and disease. Only in recent years has the medical field made a strong case for dietary treatment of some of our most severe medical problems, including heart disease.

The current interest in nutrition as treatment began with a scientific study initiated nearly forty years ago in Framingham, Massachusetts. The National Heart Institute selected that community of 28,000 people for a study that has since provided the most important, well-documented evidence of the role diet and exercise play in heart disease.

The results of the first batch of statistics, which were collected and analyzed over a period of fourteen years, documented for the first time the major risk factors for heart disease besides age and heredity: obesity, smoking, lack of physical exercise, and *high levels of cholesterol and other fats in the blood*.

The Framingham study continues today, and many more studies have sprung from this early work, linking nutrition to many of our more common ailments. It is now generally accepted that diet can play an important role in countering high blood pressure, heart disease, and some cancers.

Ironically, however, little work has been done on the effect of diet on GI diseases. Diet—the first thing people think about when they suffer digestive symptoms—is also the last thing most people, including some physicians, know anything about. We are so confused about the effect of diet on the GI tract that until very recently, doctors believed that people suffering with certain GI disorders such as IBS or diverticulosis should consume a very low-fiber diet— almost the exact opposite of what we now know to be true. Even gastroenterologists, who specialize in digestive disease, are often poorly trained in diet and nutrition. Physicians treat GI symptoms, if they treat them with diet at all, with general "tips": "Eat more fiber," or "Stay away from fatty foods." It is up to the patient to figure out how to apply this advice. This means that most fail to take advantage of new advances in diet therapy, which could greatly improve symptoms.

Some of us follow spartan diets in an attempt to reduce symptoms. Others eat foods that actually make the condition worse, or resign themselves to suffering in silence. Many people with chronic heartburn, for example, never know which foods cause the stomach to produce more acid or allow the acid to back up into the esophagus. Many people suffer from bloating, belching, or flatulence without knowing exactly which foods produce excessive gas. Others suffer unnecessarily from diarrhea, constipation, or ulcer attacks. Hundreds of thousands of people walk around with packets of antacid in their pockets at all times.

Yet a logical way to treat GI disorders is by diet. GI problems are aggravated by what we eat because food comes into direct contact with the GI tract. If the wrong food causes the problem, the right foods may solve the problem, or at least help.

The main reason doctors have been slow to recommend diet therapy is that it's complicated and hard for both physician and patient. Each patient with a GI disorder has a slightly different problem. There are many different kinds of disorders, and each has its own set of food responses. Different parts of the GI system react to different foods, and some foods affect the digestive tract in more than one site. As a result, it's common for people to have multiple GI problems. For example, a person with IBS, which affects the lower GI tract, may also suffer from upper GI symptoms, including gas pains, nausea, and heartburn. Even those of us experienced in nutritional therapy may have trouble designing a menu plan that offers good nutrition and at the same time detours around dangerous foods for every patient.

For these reasons, a comprehensive nutritional program to relieve many common GI problems is a difficult undertaking. There are hundreds of weight loss books and dozens of heart disease diets—but no single GI program.

The Self-Help Nutritional Program

In my GI practice at the Jefferson Digestive Disease Service at Thomas Jefferson University Hospital, I used to design (with the help of dietitians) an individual nutritional program for each patient—a time-consuming process. I realized that we could help many more people if we could come up with one program that almost everyone could follow.

We began by listing all the common gastrointestinal disorders and their primary symptoms. We then identified the foods and eating habits associated with each symptom. We soon saw that many of the same factors were involved with most troublesome symptoms. We culled the lists and finally isolated the six main culprits, factors responsible for a long list of symptoms.

Applying the latest nutritional research to these six diverse factors, we turned them into nutritional principles. These principles, in turn, became the foundation of a nutritional program that almost all of our GI patients could use to help themselves. It is a program designed to treat the full spectrum of common digestive disorders, from heartburn to constipation to gas to irritable bowel syndrome. It can also help prevent diverticulitis, appendicitis, hemorrhoids, and gallstones; help heal ulcers and prevent ulcer recurrence; help conquer obesity; and may lessen the likelihood of developing bowel cancer.

The six principles of the program are:

High fiber
Low fat
Low lactose
Low spice
Low gas-forming legumes
Low calories

The six principles have been incorporated into a Two-Week Master Program. Each recipe in the Master Program incorporates all six principles, and is precisely calculated to fit the nutritional specifications of the program. Each has been analyzed for macronutrient content, fiber, and calories. These recipes are based on the latest, most reliable scientific information evaluated by the Division of Gastroenterology and Department of Nutrition and Dietetics of Thomas Jefferson University Hospital.

The initial Two-Week Master Program is for everyone. After that, you can continue to repeat the Master Program, interchanging the recipes with any that appear in Part Eight of this book, or you can adapt your own recipes, using the six concepts of the program described in Part Five.

All of the recipes in *Gastrointestinal Health* were developed and tested by Cheryl Clifford Marco, R.D., manager of the hospital's outpatient nutritional counseling service, and a superb recipe writer. Each menu is designed to be easy on your digestive tract while offering flavor and variety.

This Self-Help Nutritional Program is a breakthrough in the treatment of digestive problems because it is not a one-note theory. It doesn't depend on drugs or on severe restriction of many foods. It is a high-fiber, low-fat, totally balanced diet that works in harmony with your digestive tract. It takes into account your appetite and your cravings for "comfort" foods. It also regulates the delicate biochemical balance between the brain and the digestive system so that you feel satisfied and gratified. It recognizes that foods are chemicals and that certain ratios must be maintained to soothe the digestive system, satisfy hunger, and meet nutritional needs.

Immediate Help

Learning how to treat your GI problem properly with diet does not mean blindly following a nutritional regimen for years in the hope that it is helping you. Rather it means that your symptoms are almost immediately relieved. This quick response is rarely seen with other chronic ailments that have a dietary component. For instance, diet has no direct effect on the symptoms of coronary artery disease. Eating fatty foods does not cause chest pain, nor will avoiding fatty foods alleviate chest pain. In the long run (twenty to thirty years), if you eat a heart-healthy diet you may avoid clogged arteries and you may live longer, but at the time you're eating it you can't tell that it's helping you.

Nevertheless, in addition to quick relief of GI symptoms, the longterm benefits of changing your diet can be impressive: fewer incapacitating attacks; help in controlling serious diseases such as diverticulitis; and, over years, help in the prevention of colon cancer. Such a preventive approach now could spare much grief in the future.

The Self-Help Nutritional Program makes it easy for you to change your eating habits. The initial Two-Week Master Program will prove to you just how beneficial a change in diet can be for your symptoms. After that, it is up to you to make the program work by incorporating each of the six principles into your daily meals. Relief of symptoms will be your greatest motivator: if you go back to your old habits, the symptoms will quickly return.

Because you will continue to feel well, you may soon forget what it was like to wake up every day with nausea, or to strain every time you went to the bathroom, or to have burning pain in your chest at night when you were trying to sleep. If you start slipping on the diet and begin to eat indiscriminately again, your symptoms could recur in a hurry. The GI complaints we're talking about are "diet responsive," which means that they are not usually permanently cured. So your symptoms will be your own built-in motivators.

The goal of this book is to help you minimize your dependence on drugs and maximize your control over your own health. Just as new information about the effect of nutrition on disease has steered potential heart-disease patients away from coronary bypass operations, the goal of the program is to reduce your GI symptoms without drugs whenever possible. This is a new way of thinking about treating GI problems. And not only is it good for your GI symptoms, it's good for your heart, good for your blood pressure, good for your blood sugar, and good for your cholesterol count. By all modern nutritional standards, it would be difficult to devise a healthier diet regimen.

Finally, you have the upper hand over your digestive problems. This is a program to live with; the only lifetime diet you should need. Rigid self-discipline is not central to the program. When we speak of a high-fiber, low-fat diet, we're not talking about eating bagfuls of crude bran. We are speaking of shifting the ratio of fat to fiber and fat to carbohydrates, lowering the one, while raising the other.

Dietary therapy for gastrointestinal disorders has been dramatically effective for scores of patients, some who have suffered for years from GI complaints that responded to no other therapy. For many people, following the principles of the program is enough to relieve all digestive symptoms; flare-ups occur rarely if at all. For those with serious underlying disease, the Self-Help Nutritional Program can be used as an adjunct to a drug therapy program prescribed by your physician. In these instances, following the program's principles may allow you to reduce the amount of medication you take and gain a greater measure of control over your problem.

Whether you've been plagued by GI symptoms for years and nothing has ever helped, or whether your ailment is so minor that you think you can live with it, you should try a dietary approach. Dietary management of GI problems really works for real people. If you suffer from any common digestive problem, this may be the program you've been waiting for.

Part One

━━━━━━━━━━━━━━━━━━━━━━━━━━━━━━━━━━━━━

Gastrointestinal Health

1

The Self-Help Nutritional Program: A Healing Diet

*T*he science of nutrition is a changing field, and different concepts become fashionable almost weekly. New reports seem to contradict what has gone before and, invariably, new fads based on incomplete data emerge.

Amid the confusion, American eating habits have undergone profound changes. Today, one-third of our meals are consumed outside the home; when we do eat at home, we often resort to prepared convenience foods. All of us have to struggle harder to maintain nutritional balance, and the struggle is more difficult for people with GI disorders who are subject to severe and debilitating symptoms.

Many become fixated on their next meal, worrying in advance about their reactions. They know instinctively that some foods make their problems worse, but don't know how to establish a nutritional routine they can depend on. In frustration, some people end up eating almost nothing. Existing on too little food, smoking too much for oral gratification, which makes the GI disorder worse, they are often irritable and frustrated.

Double Trouble

One patient of ours was a twenty-eight-year-old ballet dancer who constantly yo-yoed on and off weight-loss diets to maintain a perfectly slim body. At the same time, she was under high performance stress. While still in her teens Margo began to have severe and sudden stomach cramps, followed by diarrhea; she had her first ulcer attack on her twenty-first birthday. She had suffered on and off from both problems ever since. Although Margo had taken many different drugs in an effort to control the various symptoms, she was still vulnerable to sudden, painful attacks that sometimes lasted weeks at a time. And as so commonly happens with GI patients, the foods recommended for one condition were problems for the other.

Some Myths and Facts

Here are a few more of our common misconceptions about diet and GI disorders.

Myth: A bland diet relieves ulcer symptoms. The traditional ulcer diet includes milk, cream, rice, fish, and other bland food. It was believed that eating small, tasteless meals would help ulcers heal by reducing acid secretion and setting up a buffer against stomach acid.

Fact: A diet high in milk products can actually be harmful to ulcers because milk and cream *increase* acid production in the stomach, which can delay ulcer healing. A bland diet is often a low-fiber diet. Fiber is now thought to aid ulcer healing. Fiber may also help prevent relapse of duodenal ulcers by slowing the rate at which the stomach empties. The only foods to be avoided by someone with ulcer pain are specific "Flag Foods" (see Chapter 24).

Myth: Constipation is a normal part of life, especially as you grow older, and is best treated by laxatives as needed.

Fact: Many people have become dependent on laxatives or enemas, claiming that this is the only way they can move their bowels. After long-term laxative abuse, many people develop "lazy bowel," and the bowel ceases to function normally. Stimulant laxatives also cause colicky pain by strengthening bowel contractions against dry, hard stool. For the great majority of people, the best way to treat and prevent constipation is by a high-fiber diet.

Myth: Heartburn is caused by a hiatal hernia or by eating spicy foods.

Fact: Many people with heartburn do not have hiatal hernias. And many foods that are not spicy can promote heartburn, including chocolate, tea, coffee, and fatty foods. Spicy foods by themselves will not cause inflammation of the esophagus or the stomach, but can make symptoms worse if the lining is already inflamed.

Margo came to us after a long bout of cramps and diarrhea that had left her frustrated and weak. We diagnosed her symptoms as irritable bowel syndrome, and recommended that she follow the Two-Week Master Program. We also suggested that she join a stop-smoking group because we felt certain that cigarettes were aggravating her symptoms.

Even though Margo had voluntarily sought our help, she seemed ambivalent about taking our advice. I wondered if there was something about her illness that she was keeping from me. After talking with her about her profession it became obvious that Margo liked one of the side effects of her GI disorder—it helped keep her weight down. Margo's symptoms were often so severe that she couldn't eat anything at all. She would go to parties and dinners and smoke cigarettes—but never touch a morsel of food. The cigarettes, which raised her already high rate of metabolism even further, supplied the oral gratification she missed from food.

There was another element working against any program to treat her disorder—she had a high tolerance for pain. Her profession sometimes required that she endure extreme muscle pain, and dance through periods of exhaustion. Physical suffering seemed fairly normal to her.

The magic words that finally convinced Margo to get serious about the Self-Help Nutritional Program were "You can eat three meals a day on the Two-Week Program and you will not gain weight."

Margo was a hard case. Interestingly enough, however, once she "got" it—once she accepted the fact that she could eat real food and be free from pain without gaining weight—it was a snap for her to start the program and stick to it. She was so naturally disciplined that she thought nothing of following the regimen.

One element of the program especially appealed to her. Even though the Two-Week Master Program is recommended for most common digestive disorders, each problem has its own set of "triggers"— foods or other factors that make the disorder flare—because specific foods irritate specific parts of the GI system. We call these triggers *Flag Foods*. When we developed the Self-Help Nutritional Program we identified Flag Foods for each GI disorder. (Lists of Flag Foods for each disorder are given in Chapter 24.)

Knowing which Flag Foods affect your particular problem(s) lets you fine-tune the Self-Help Nutritional Program to your individual needs. Some people have to be wary of only one or two Flag Foods, while others have to avoid a whole list of Flag Foods to keep their symptoms under control. Flag Foods give you an easy way to loosen or tighten the reins on the Self-Help Nutritional Program.

Margo quickly learned all of her Flag Foods. When faced with a rushed lunch hour or late-night snack after the theater she could pick out her Flag Foods and avoid them. She selected the lowest-calorie recipes from recipes low in calories to begin with, and she ate them regularly.

Margo's abdominal cramps subsided almost immediately, and she had no counterresponse from the ulcers. No one was more surprised than we were when she came in for a routine follow-up visit and told us she had stopped smoking—cold turkey. That was Margo's nature. Once she made up her mind, it was done. Ultimately, Margo became one of our greatest success stories. To date, she has gone a full year without an attack from either of her GI disorders.

*F*or some people who lead hectic lives, switching to new eating habits can seem impossible. Not everyone is as self-disciplined as Margo.

I remember George, a young trial attorney who popped antacid tablets throughout the day to try to cope with overwhelming heartburn. If he had an attack while in court he would suffer through it without the antacid because he didn't want the opposing lawyer or the jury to know he had a problem. Often his attacks occurred at night when he went to bed, especially after grabbing a late-night snack on his way home from the office.

Finally, his symptoms were nonstop, and he came for treatment. He wanted me to give him a bigger and better antacid tablet. George didn't have a clue about why he had heartburn. "I think it's because I'm a few pounds overweight," he told me. He was partly right, but there were other reasons as well.

George's life was complicated. He lived alone. He often worked around the clock, consuming chocolate shakes, hamburgers, and French fries at his desk in the middle of the night. If he had time off he went out partying with his friends. If George knew where his kitchen was he gave no sign of it.

I explained the mechanisms that caused his heartburn and told him there was no way to control his attacks in the courtroom or in the middle of the night—short of chronic heavy doses of drugs—unless he changed his destructive eating habits. I explained the principles of the Self-Help Nutritional Program, and also gave him a list of the Flag Foods known to aggravate heartburn.

George seemed overwhelmed by the prospect of these changes, but I insisted he give the program a try. George's mother helped him get started by going grocery shopping for him and stocking his kitchen pantry with enough high-fiber, low-fat foods to last a month. She prepared some of the entrees recommended in the Two-Week Master Program and put them in his freezer. Then she taped his list of Flag Foods to the door of his refrigerator. Under this she added a hand-lettered poster citing one of George's worst heartburn-provoking habits. It said, Do NOT EAT BEFORE GOING TO BED. She then browbeat her son into trying the first week of the Two-Week Master Program.

Within forty-eight hours George felt 100 percent better. Without ever resorting to drug therapy and taking only occasional antacids, George felt immediate relief of his symptoms. By the end of the week his roll of Tums was gathering dust on top of his dresser. His excellent response was typical of the remarkable improvement that can be achieved with proper dietary treatment of heartburn.

George's mother wasn't in the mood to baby him forever, however. After the first week, George had to manage the nutritional program on

GI Problems the Self-Help Nutritional Program Can Help

Condition	Helps Prevent	Heals	Helps Control or Reduce
Appendicitis	X		
Colon cancer	X		
Constipation	X	X	X
Coronary artery disease	X		
Crohn's disease			X
Diabetes	X		X
Diverticulitis	X		
Diverticulosis	X		X
Esophagitis	X	X	X
Gallbladder disease	X		X
Gallstones	X		X
Heartburn	X	X	X
Hemorrhoids	X	X	X
High cholesterol	X		X
Hypertension	X		X
IBS			X
Obesity	X	X	X
Ulcers	X		X

his own. Fortunately, the guidelines and recipes for the program are so simple that even George could incorporate them into his hectic life. One year later, he is still following the program. He slips from time to time, but renewal of the old heartburn symptoms quickly puts him back on track. Overall, George says the program isn't nearly as difficult as he expected. For him, the rewards far outweigh the effort needed to change his eating habits.

Even if you think "culinary" is a foreign word, you can manage the Self-Help Nutritional Program. Even if you're like George, who would rather have a magic pill to make it all go away, you can get with the program and personally take control of your health.

The Self-Help Nutritional Program lends itself particularly to the treatment of the most common GI problems—heartburn, peptic ulcers, chronic pancreatitis, gallbladder disease, gas, constipation, mild diarrhea, hemorrhoids, IBS, and diverticulosis.*

The program is designed for people who already have significant digestive symptoms, which means that it is much more than a healthy diet. It is a *healing* diet. It is naturally low in calories. It avoids excessive caffeine and keeps alcohol to a minimum. It tells you to stop smoking because smoking makes most GI disorders worse. Most importantly, the Self-Help Nutritional Program shows you how to identify the Flag Foods that trigger GI problems in *you*.

---

* The diet is not recommended for people with acute diverticulitis and moderate to severe inflammatory bowel disease (Crohn's disease; ulcerative colitis) unless directed by a physician.

2   *How the GI Tract Works*

The digestive tract is a long, intricate system that comprises many separate organs, each performing different functions. To successfully treat a GI problem with diet means understanding the complex workings of the gastrointestinal system, and how the food you eat affects it.

The body runs itself by absorbing nutrients processed by the digestive system. At the center of the digestive system is the alimentary canal, or gastrointestinal tract, which travels from mouth to anus in 30 feet of tightly packed coils. From beginning to end, food is ingested and processed, nutrients are absorbed, and residue is propelled to the end of the tract and finally eliminated.

Your GI tract will digest about 23,000 pounds of solid food in your lifetime, which makes it a very efficient, hard-working system. It takes between twelve and fifteen hours for a single morsel of food to be fully processed, although it can take much longer, depending on the kind of morsel it is. Meat goes slower, grain goes faster.

From top to bottom, the GI tract is made up of the mouth, pharynx, esophagus, stomach, small intestine, and large intestine.

Mouth, Pharynx, and Esophagus

Digestion begins in the mouth. When you chew, salivary glands in the cheek and glands at the back of the tongue produce enzymes that break the food into fragments. Specific enzymes break down carbohydrates and fats respectively.

When you swallow, complex controlling mechanisms within the pharynx, the common passageway for food and air, ensure that food goes into the esophagus, instead of into the windpipe (trachea).

The esophagus is the passageway between the mouth and the stomach. The delicate lining of the esophagus is the site of heartburn, the most common GI complaint. Swallowed food quickly passes through the esophagus into the stomach, where it is temporarily stored.

Stomach

The stomach is a large, tough organ with three layers of muscle, running up and down, across, and crosswise. As these muscles contract, the food mixture is churned up. The stomach adds quantities of digestive enzymes and strong hydrochloric acid to the churning mixture, which break it down into complex nutrients. The stomach lining normally withstands the noxious acid by forming a mucus barrier against it. If acid production is excessive, however, or if the barrier is weak, the stomach lining may be eroded. The result is an ulcer.

Although a few substances, such as aspirin, may enter the bloodstream directly through the stomach walls, most food is stored here until contractions of the smooth muscle wall pump it into the small intestine. It may take between two and four hours or longer for an average-sized meal to be pumped into the small intestine. Even when the stomach is empty, the muscles continue their steady pumping action. The wavelike contractions, called peristalsis, create the familiar pangs that signal "hunger" to the brain. The growling sound made by the continuous contractions tends to be louder when the stomach is empty. Anxiety causes an even louder noise because the smooth muscle is responsive to stress.

Small Intestine

Most of the serious business of digestion and absorption occurs in the long, narrow, small intestine. The food mixture first enters the duodenum, another likely place for ulcers to develop because the mixture is still acidic. The major work of digestion begins here with action from certain hormones. One hormone, called cholecystokinin, or CCK, draws in bile from the gallbladder to make fat more digestible. This same hormone also draws juices from the pancreas to calm the acidity left in the food mixture and to aid digestion of fat, protein, and carbohydrates.

The food mixture slows down as it travels along the small intestine to allow time for refined processing and absorption. Proteins are split by various enzymes into individual amino acids; carbohydrate becomes simple sugar; and fat becomes glycerol and fatty acid. In this form, food can be absorbed by the body. Millions of tiny fingerlike projections called villi line the interior of the small intestine, increasing its surface area. As the nutrients pass by, the villi pick them out and transport them into the bloodstream.

The digestive system now begins to interact with another body system, the circulatory system. Nutrients travel through the bloodstream to the liver, a giant chemical factory that is the key organ of human metabolism.

GASTROINTESTINAL TRACT
 1. Hypopharynx (throat)
 2. Upper esophageal sphincter
 3. Esophagus
 4. Lower esophageal sphincter
 5. Stomach
 6. Pylorus (pyloric valve or channel)
 7. Duodenum
 8. Pancreas
 9. Liver
10. Gallbladder
11. Common bile duct
12. Spleen
13. Small intestine (jejunum)
14. Small intestine (ileum)
15. Terminal ileum
16. Cecum
17. Appendix
18. Ascending (right) colon
19. Transverse colon
20. Descending (left) colon
21. Sigmoid colon
22. Diverticuli
23. Rectum
24. Anus

The liver works around the clock to secrete bile, make various proteins, and remove toxic substances from ingested food. Blood that has circulated through the liver is ready to be used as fuel by body cells. If the liver fails, the body dies.

With the exception of most fats, all nutrients enter the bloodstream via the liver. Most digested fats are absorbed by the villi and shipped to the lymphatic system, where they are then returned to the bloodstream.

Large Intestine

After all possible nutrients have been absorbed through the walls of the small intestine, a watery mix of undigested fiber is left. This residue of fecal matter is propelled toward the large intestine, or colon. The large intestine, which is much shorter (only 3 feet, compared to the 20-foot length of the small intestine) and fatter than the small intestine, absorbs excess water from the fiber residue and stores the feces. Eventually the feces are evacuated by the last portion of the colon, the rectum, and discharged through a muscular canal called the anus.

Besides fiber, feces also contain large quantities of living and dead bacteria, along with debris shed by the lining of the intestines. People who consume highly refined, low-fiber foods may have little actual fiber residue in the feces. Those who eat substantial quantities of vegetables and grains will have much more residue.

Many digestive problems arise here in the lower GI tract. Diverticulosis, a condition in which little ballooned sacs of intestinal membrane have been forced outward by high pressure, is one of the most common lower GI tract disorders. Appendicitis, although not a digestive disorder per se, is another problem that arises here. The appendix is a fingerlike projection hanging from the large intestine that helps certain animals digest plant matter. In humans, the appendix is probably useless. However, when it collects bacteria and undigested food, it can swell up and may even burst, which is a life-threatening situation. People who consume a high-fiber diet are much less likely to develop appendicitis. The reason is that fiber keeps the food moving through the intestines, and this regular, fairly rapid transit prevents the accumulation of trapped and stagnant bacteria.

Colon cancer, second in prevalence only to lung cancer when statistics for men and women are combined, is another potentially dangerous condition that arises in the lower GI tract.

Despite its complexity, the digestive system works in a remarkably smooth fashion for most people most of the time. When all is well with the GI tract, the only thing you have to think about is eating when you are hungry and moving your bowels when pressure builds up in the rectum. You may hear your stomach growl when you are hungry or hear gurgling as peristaltic contractions propel food along the GI tract, but you should not actually *feel* these actions. Digesting and absorbing food should be as effortless and comfortable as breathing. At least that's what nature intended.

How Civilization Has Altered Digestion

In our evolutionary past it's unlikely that our ancestors ever had many of the types of digestive problems we frequently experience today. Cave dwellers and some of their descendants had cast-iron stomachs, which processed anything put into them. Our earliest ancestors ate nuts, seeds, roots, and wild plants. They brought every animal that ever moved to the dinner table—game and birds, as well as ants and bees, grubs and worms, snakes and mice. As they became agriculturists and began to grow their own plants and raise domestic livestock, some built villages along the coastlines and rivers and added quantities of fish and shellfish to their diets. Our prehistoric food pattern may not have been ideal in every respect, but it served the human body reasonably well because it contained extensive nutrients and minimal pollutants.

In different cultures, in different parts of the world, at different times in history, humans have eaten a startlingly wide array of materials. Joseph Addison, who lived in the sixteenth century, observed, "Every animal, but man, keeps to one dish. Man falls upon everything that comes in his way; not the smallest fruit or excrescence of the earth, scarce a berry or a mushroom can escape him."

One thing this wide variety of foods had in common was that it came in its natural state, stems and roots, husks and skins, seeds and pits. Once inside the GI tract it required quite a bit of processing to digest. Over several million years the human body developed a highly efficient processing plant that could squeeze every possible nutrient from the items we ate. Anything left over after the processing plant did its job was efficiently eliminated through the colon.

Then a sudden drastic change occurred in our diet, with no time allowed for evolutionary adjustment. A real machine took over the processing job. With the development of the rolling mill in the nineteenth century, the bran and germ of cereal grains was removed in the processing of flour. Sugar was processed from cane, oil was processed from seeds. Bread consumption fell by two-thirds.

Losing Nutrition

Food went through a sudden evolution of its own, and began to arrive on store shelves in small boxes instead of bushel baskets. Soon processed foods turned into Twinkies and Oreos, and "junk foods" proliferated in both supermarkets and restaurants. The small amount of fiber remaining in foods was lost.

Of all the many weird and spectacular creatures and plants that humans had consumed, none ever came close to resembling a chocolate shake or a hamburger bun topped with a fatty beef patty, processed cheese, mayonnaise, pickles, and catsup. None ever looked like soda pop or a sugar-coated donut with custard and jelly filling. Even our remarkable adaptability could not deal with the steady stream of refined sugar, bleached white flour, hydrogenated fat, and salt that poured into the typical American diet. Even rats could not survive on white bread, which was (and is) the most commonly eaten food in America.

The change in our eating habits was as if we suddenly started to pour paste through a highly complex engine. Our GI engine became clogged and sluggish. Functioning was impaired. Constipation became common, and caused much unnecessary discomfort and pain associated with hemorrhoids, diverticulosis, and varicose veins. The incidence of duodenal ulcers increased, probably due to stress.

The incidence of appendicitis doubled. The appendix tends to collect debris when there is not enough bulk to keep residue moving rapidly through the colon. This leads to clogging and infection. One study that analyzed the diets of 135 children with appendicitis and 212 children without it, showed that children who consumed low-fiber diets were twice as likely to develop appendicitis.

At the same time, our consumption of alcohol, tobacco, and caffeine increased. In an era when the body needed more nutrients to fight environmental toxins, stress, drugs, alcohol, and tobacco, we were getting even less.

The radical shift in diet and environment over the past hundred years is directly related to the GI ailments that we face today. Everyone of us has a GI upset sometimes, and many of us—in fact, 80 million of us—have chronic symptoms.

3   *What Your Symptoms Mean*

*P*ressure, burning pain, and spasm are the primary symptoms of digestive disorders that you may *feel*. Other symptoms that you may experience, but don't necessarily feel, are constipation, diarrhea, bleeding, belching, flatulence, and weight loss.

Although the range of symptoms appears limited, the number of possible disorders is long. It's not always easy to identify a GI disorder by the symptom it produces. Nor is the degree of pain always an indication of the severity of the disorder. Some serious disorders produce relatively little pain, while minor problems can create pain out of proportion to their importance.

You may mistakenly believe you have one kind of GI problem, and really have another. Or more than one. Spasms, for example, can occur anywhere along the digestive tract. When spasm occurs in the esophagus it is often indistinguishable from a heart attack. Spasm of the esophagus may also cause difficulty in swallowing. It can occur suddenly without cause, or in response to cold or hot liquids, acid reflux, or stress.

A spasm further down the GI tract may produce a sharp pain in the abdomen that makes you double over. Spasm here may be associated with diarrhea, blockage of the bowel, gallstones, or irritable bowel syndrome (IBS).

So, location of the symptom can sometimes help determine the cause. Burning pains usually involve the upper GI tract. Burning may be felt in the middle of the chest just beneath the breastbone (heartburn) or in the upper abdomen (ulcers or pancreatitis).

Feelings of abdominal distension and cramping are symptoms often involving the middle and lower GI tract (small and large intestines). Irritable bowel syndrome, diverticulitis, and excessive intestinal gas are typical problems that arise in this region.

Note: Unexplained weight loss, difficulty swallowing, rectal bleeding, frequent urge to move your bowels, and recent onset of constipation are symptoms that should receive prompt attention and diagnosis from your physician as they may be signs of serious disease.

What Your Symptoms Mean

Symptom	Location	Possible Cause	Helped by the Self-Help Nutritional Program?	
			Yes	No
Burning pain	Below breastbone	Heartburn	X	
	Pit of stomach	Peptic ulcers	X	
		Pancreatitis	X	
	Anus	Hemorrhoids	X	
Spasm or cramping	Below breastbone	Esophageal spasm	X*	
		Heart attack		X
	Right upper abdomen	Gallstones	X	
	Pit of stomach	Stress	X	
		Gas	X	
	Around umbilicus	Gas	X	
		Constriction of blood vessel		X
		Bowel obstruction		X
		Early appendicitis		X
	Lower abdomen	IBS	X	
		Constipation	X	
		Diarrhea	X	
	Right lower abdomen	Ileitis (Crohn's disease)	X†	
		Appendicitis		X
	Left lower abdomen	Diverticulosis	X	
		Diverticulitis		X

* Often helpful in preventing triggers of spasm (acid reflux, spicy foods).
† Often helpful in mild cases; can be contraindicated in severe Crohn's disease. Always consult your doctor before starting the Self-Help Nutritional Program if you have Crohn's disease.

Find Your Gut Reaction Quotient

If you suffer from GI distress but have never had your symptoms properly diagnosed by a physician it is important to do so before embarking on the Self-Help Nutritional Program. The program is a healthy diet for almost everyone, but digestive symptoms can sometimes signal serious disease that requires medical therapy. Relying solely on self-diagnosis is risky because symptoms of a mild disorder such as irritable bowel syndrome may be identical to symptoms of a life-threatening disease such as bowel cancer. Only your physician can make a specific diagnosis of your GI problem. Often diagnosis can be made during a regular office visit, but sometimes further tests are required.

The following quiz can help you inventory your GI complaints. Many GI sufferers ultimately come to accept as normal levels of distress that healthier individuals would find unacceptable. The quiz will let you gain a sense of control over what may seem to be an escalating range of symptoms. Answering yes to any of the questions listed below means that you should see your physician for specific diagnosis. If the diagnosis falls within the range of the common digestive disorders discussed in this book, you are a good candidate for the Self-Help Nutritional Program.

1 Do you frequently have a sour taste in your mouth when you lie down or bend over? (This means acid has refluxed from the stomach up the esophagus to your mouth.)

2 Do you occasionally regurgitate undigested food? (You may have a defective sphincter [valve] at the end of your esophagus, which allows gastric contents to reflux back up into the esophagus.)

3 Do you frequently wake up in the middle of the night coughing? (This could be caused by acid reflux being aspirated into the lungs when you lie down. If you have this particular symptom your physician will first rule out a heart or lung problem.)

4 Do certain foods such as citrus juice burn on the way down to your stomach? (Burning indicates that the esophagus is inflamed, usually caused by acid reflux. If you are immune compromised in any way—if you take drugs that suppress the immune system or if you have advanced cancer or AIDS—your physician will first rule out infection of the esophagus caused by yeast or herpes simplex.)

5   Do you experience heartburn, that burning feeling underneath the breastbone, more than twice a month?

6   Do you frequently belch? (If the belching occurs because you are swallowing air, therapy such as counseling or relaxation techniques can help treat the underlying cause of anxiety. If the belching is caused by reflux problems, the Self-Help Nutritional Program is for you.)

7   Do you have trouble swallowing solids or liquids? (Your esophagus may be obstructed or it may not be contracting properly. See your physician before embarking on any dietary changes.)

8   Do you get a burning or gnawing pain in the upper abdomen between the breastbone and the navel? (This could be a symptom of gastric ulcers, gastritis [inflammation of the stomach lining], duodenal ulcers, duodenitis [inflammation of the duodenum], or pancreatitis. Much less commonly this symptom is associated with cancer of the stomach.)

9   Do you ever get black, tarry bowel movements? (You may have a bleeding ulcer. See your doctor immediately.)

10   Do you feel full right after you start eating? (This so-called early satiety may indicate significant stomach problems, especially if it is recent in onset. See your doctor as soon as possible.)

11   Have you recently had an episode of waxing and waning sharp or dull pain just below your rib cage on the right side? (This symptom suggests gallstones. After correct diagnosis, the Self-Help Nutritional Program can help relieve symptoms.)

12   Do you have a yellowish tinge to your skin or the whites of your eyes (best seen in natural sunlight)? This may be associated with itching, dark amber urine, and light clay-colored stools. (These symptoms may mean you have liver disease or your bile duct system is blocked. See your doctor right away.)

13   Do you have frequent episodes of pain in both sides of the lower abdomen? (If your doctor says you have IBS, start the Self-Help Nutritional Program.)

14   Do you have frequent episodes of pain in the left lower abdomen? (If your doctor says you have IBS or diverticulosis, start the Self-Help Nutritional Program. If the diagnosis is *diverticulitis*, meaning that the little pouches, or diverticula, are inflamed, postpone the program until you have received appropriate medical treatment for the acute inflammation.)

15 Do you have frequent episodes of pain in your right lower abdomen? (See your doctor. You may have appendicitis, ovarian cysts, or ileitis [Crohn's disease]. If your physician rules out these conditions and makes a diagnosis of IBS, you can start the Self-Help Nutritional Program.)

16 Do you have a history of chronic diarrhea and rectal bleeding? (You could have inflammatory bowel disease [ulcerative colitis or Crohn's disease], colon polyps, hemorrhoids, or dysentery [bacterial infection of the bowel]. See your doctor.)

17 Do you have a long history of loose stools, constipation, or constipation alternating with diarrhea? (This is a likely case of IBS, which responds well to the Self-Help Nutritional Program. If this is a new symptom, however, it's important to see your doctor for diagnosis.)

18 Have you recently become constipated? (This could signal a tumor blocking the colon, especially if you are over forty years old. Other possible causes of constipation are recent travel, irritable bowel syndrome, and side effects of drugs such as Procardia and Carafate. See your doctor as soon as possible.)

19 Are your stools pencil-thin in shape? (Again, this could reflect a blockage of the colon by a tumor. See your doctor.)

20 Do you constantly feel the need to move your bowels, even if you can't, or even if you've just had a bowel movement? (This symptom, called tenesmus, is sometimes caused by partial blockages of the colon. See your doctor right away.)

21 Do you experience frequent episodes of flatulence that bother you? (Some flatulence is normal, but some people have excessive flatulence. The Self-Help Nutritional Program can help. See Chapters 10 and 24.)

22 Are you losing weight without trying? (Unexplained weight loss is associated with several potentially serious diseases. See your doctor as soon as possible.)

23 Do you suffer from hemorrhoids or anal fissures? (The Self-Help Nutritional Program can definitely help you, but your doctor will first want to make certain that you do not have an associated colon problem.)

24 Do you notice blood on the surface of the stools, in the toilet bowl, or on the toilet paper when you wipe? (This usually means you have hemorrhoids or a fissure. Occasionally, inflammatory bowel disease confined to the rectum [proctitis] can cause this symptom. See your doctor.)

25 Do you notice blood mixed in the stool? (This usually means that the blood has entered the stool higher up in the colon. You could have a polyp, tumor, bleeding diverticula, or inflammatory bowel disease. See your doctor.)

26 Do you have itching around the anus? (You could have hemorrhoids, but pinworms is another possibility, especially if you have small children. See your doctor.)

How a Doctor Diagnoses Your Problem

On the initial visit the physician usually makes a working diagnosis based on the most likely cause of your symptoms. Often there is also a "differential diagnosis," a list of different possibilities that could also account for your symptoms. For example, if you are a young woman with long-standing constipation occasionally alternating with diarrhea and cramps in the lower abdomen, but no sign of fever, weight loss, or blood in the stool, then the most likely diagnosis is irritable bowel syndrome. But other possibilities would include inflammatory bowel disease (ulcerative colitis or Crohn's disease), bowel cancer, endometriosis, and several other less likely possibilities.

Your physician may recommend treatment based on the symptoms alone. Or, if there is a possibility of serious underlying disease, he or she is likely to carry out one or more GI tests to clearly pinpoint the diagnosis and rule out other diseases.

Here are some of the common tests used to evaluate the GI tract.

Upper GI Series (Barium Swallow). You swallow a solution of barium, and a radiologist uses a fluoroscope connected to a TV monitor to observe the progress of the contrast medium through your digestive tract. The radiologist takes individual x-rays to review. The upper GI series examines the esophagus, stomach, and the first part of the small intestine (duodenum). The test may also include a small bowel follow-through, performed immediately afterward, to examine the entire length of the small intestine. Sometimes the procedure is carried out using "double contrast" media, meaning that you also swallow tablets to release gas in your stomach. The gas helps show the stomach lining in greater detail.

The upper GI series is performed if you have one or more of the following symptoms: difficulty swallowing, history of ulcer, abdominal pain relieved by eating, pain within an hour of eating, heartburn, gastrointestinal bleeding. It can help diagnose narrowing of the esophagus, inflammation or strictures of the esophagus, hiatal hernia, or spasms. It can identify gastric and duodenal ulcers or tumors. The small bowel follow-through may reveal ileitis (Crohn's disease).

Sometimes additional studies are needed to directly visualize the upper GI tract (see below).

Endoscopy. Endoscopy allows direct visualization of the upper GI tract. The endoscope, a long thin tube with a viewing lens and a lighted tip, is inserted through your mouth (after appropriate sedation) and then gently advanced down into the esophagus, stomach, and duodenum.

This allows the physician to look directly into the upper GI tract for ulcers, inflammation, tumors, or bleeding. Tissue samples can be collected for biopsy through the endoscope. Polyps can be removed, and bleeding can often be stopped by applying an electrical current to the site (electrocautery).

Bernstein Test. Sometimes this test is used to distinguish cardiac pain from heartburn. You swallow a small tube so that one end rests near the end of the esophagus. The physician first infuses saltwater through the tube into the esophagus, and then follows with a weak solution of hydrochloric acid. If you feel a typical burning sensation in the chest only with the acid solution, but feel nothing unusual with the saline solution, the test is considered positive for reflux esophagitis.

pH Probe. A more recent development is the pH Probe, a thin tube inserted into the esophagus that can measure the pH of acid in the esophagus over a twelve- to twenty-four-hour period. The pH is analyzed over a day while you are working, eating, and sleeping, to determine how many episodes of reflux you have and how long each lasts. The occurrence of symptoms can then be matched with your activity at that particular time.

Electrocardiogram. Sometimes an electrocardiogram (EKG) is done to rule out heart problems and distinguish heartburn from angina.

Lower GI Series. After an overnight fast and a bowel-cleansing regimen that includes laxatives and enemas, barium is placed by enema into the colon and x-rays are taken. This test is used to detect polyps, inflammation of the colon, and colon cancer. The test may be single (barium only) or double contrast (barium and air).

Flexible Sigmoidoscopy. The flexible sigmoidoscope is a 2-foot-long tube containing a powerful light source that works on the principle of fiberoptics, or as a video camera. The instrument allows a physician to directly examine the lining of the rectum and a portion of the lower colon. The procedure is used to investigate unexplained rectal bleeding, change in bowel habits, or rectal pain. Sigmoidoscopy is also used to evaluate abnormalities found on barium x-rays, and to monitor progress of polyps or inflammatory bowel disease. The physician can also remove small polyps and tissue samples through the sigmoidoscope.

Colonoscopy. This procedure is similar to sigmoidoscopy, but the entire length of the colon is investigated. It is most often used to evaluate unexplained blood in the stool, abdominal pain, persistent diarrhea, or polyps found on barium x-rays. Sometimes colonoscopy is used to determine the type and extent of inflammatory bowel disease (ulcerative colitis and Crohn's disease) and to screen patients who are known to be at high risk for colon cancer, such as patients with a long history of ulcerative colitis or a family history of colon cancer.

Gallbladder Studies. The purpose of a gallbladder series is to observe the gallbladder in action. It may be carried out using a contrast medium and x-rays, or by ultrasound. The idea is first to prevent the gallbladder from contracting by depriving the digestive tract of fats through fasting; then to take x-rays or an ultrasound of the gallbladder at rest. Afterward, you are asked to ingest fats, either through a special high-fat formula or by going out and eating a high-fat meal. The presence of fat in your digestive system causes the gallbladder to contract, and a new series of x-rays is taken at fifteen-, thirty-, and sometimes sixty-minute intervals to observe how the gallbladder responds. The tests can detect gallstones and inflammation of the gallbladder.

*I*n most cases, though, GI symptoms do not mean that you have a serious disease. There are a few serious digestive disorders that the Self-Help Nutritional Program cannot help. Most diseases of the small intestine, such as adhesions that cause kinks in the intestine, are examples. Inflammatory bowel disease, in the form of Crohn's disease or ulcerative colitis, often goes through periods of intense inflammation when a high-fiber diet may be contraindicated. These conditions require medical treatment and special dietary planning. For the most part, however, all of the disorders that follow can be improved by following the Self-Help Nutritional Program.

4

Is Your GI Disorder Psychosomatic?
The Brain-Gut Connection

Many people get the idea that their GI complaints aren't "real" because their doctor can't find any reason for their trouble.

Digestive disorders are classified as either *functional or organic.* Disorders like gastroesophageal reflux (esophagitis), inflammatory bowel disease (Crohn's disease; ulcerative colitis), and colon cancer are defined as organic. "Organic" means that the problem arises from a disease state, such as an inflamed colon or large intestine, which causes structural damage that can be detected with various tests.

For instance, when I insert a colonoscope into the colon of a patient with active ulcerative colitis, I can readily see the damage. Instead of the usual normal pinkish color, the lining of the colon is bright red, there is a sore or break in its surface, and it bleeds easily.

"Functional" means that something isn't working properly, but there is no recognizable organic or structural damage. In the case of functional GI disorders, something is amiss with the fine tuning of the system, even though the individual parts appear normal. Subtle biochemical defects may be causing the problem. Or perhaps the parts are poorly coordinated, so that the system doesn't function optimally.

Functional and organic problems may produce similar symptoms, but they may not respond to the same kind of treatment. Organic disorders, for example, often require drug therapy, along with dietary changes. Functional disorders, which are usually less dangerous, often do not respond well to drug therapy, but they may respond remarkably well to dietary change.

Many of my patients seem to be disappointed when nothing is found on the diagnostic tests and relieved when something *is* found, even when the problem is potentially serious. This seems unreasonable. I would much rather learn that my lower abdominal cramps are caused by irritable bowel syndrome than by ulcerative colitis or bowel cancer. The functional disorder is relatively harmless; the others are more serious. But many people are afraid they might be labeled as nuts, crocks, or hypochondriacs if they have a functional disorder. In truth, the functional label does not mean that your GI problem is all in your head or that you brought the symptoms on yourself.

When a patient's symptoms are evaluated and all the tests ordered come back normal, some doctors might say the symptoms are *psychosomatic*. "Psychosomatic," as the word implies, means that in some way the mind or brain is causing dysfunction of the body. This may imply to the patient that the doctor feels the problem is not "real." That's why doctors don't use the term very much anymore. Although there is little evidence that the mind can actually cause disease, it can certainly make preexisting GI conditions worse. The so-called brain-gut connection is very real.

There are nerves that travel from the brain to the esophagus, stomach, gallbladder, pancreas, small intestine, and colon. That is why just looking at or smelling food can stimulate stomach and intestinal contractions, as well as stomach acid and pancreatic enzyme secretion.

It's no wonder that in periods of stress, when nervous discharge is on overload, excessive gastrointestinal motility can cause cramps, excessive acid secretion, and burning abdominal pain in certain predisposed individuals.

Many people can handle stress without experiencing gut-wrenching problems, but if you have irritable bowel syndrome, your threshold for experiencing intestinal pain may be lower. Likewise, if you were born with extra acid secreting cells in the stomach, psychic stress may cause such an outpouring of acid that inflammation of the stomach lining results.

In fact, it appears that the brain has an important effect not only on functional bowel problems, but organic problems as well. Stress can make symptoms worse in organic disorders such as inflammatory bowel disease, peptic ulcer disease, and gastroesophageal reflux disease. Studies have even shown that stress and mental attitude can have a negative effect on survival from cancer.

So don't be too upset if your doctor can't find an organic cause for your symptoms, and don't worry if your symptoms act up under periods of stress. Having a functional problem or having a psychosomatic component to your disorder should not carry a stigma.

One of our patients, a thirty-two-year-old woman named Sara, suffered from severe cramps in the lower abdomen. She had pain at various times during the month, and it did not appear to be associated with her menstrual periods. Sara did notice a correlation between her symptoms and episodes of stress in her job selling computer software. The gut-twisting cramps were often followed by severe bouts of diarrhea; then she might have several days of constipation. The constipation made her feel bloated and she said her waistline seemed to increase by two or three inches. Her symptoms became so severe at times that they interfered with her job and her social life.

Sara had been to several doctors who performed many tests, including a barium enema, upper GI series, sigmoidoscopy, and pelvic exam with ultrasound. All test results were normal. According to the tests there was nothing wrong with Sara. One doctor told her that her symptoms were psychosomatic. Another finally told her that she had a condition called irritable bowel syndrome (IBS), or spastic colon, for which there is no identifiable cause. IBS affects almost three out of every ten young women. It isn't a life-threatening problem, but unfortunately drugs rarely work to control symptoms.

Since IBS appears to be stress related, Sara's doctor had suggested she relax more. Good advice, but not always easy to follow. Sara didn't know how to relax. And she resented the doctor's implication that she was causing her own problem. But she tried. She went on a European vacation and experienced IBS symptoms almost every day she was away. Catching trains and planes, moving from one hotel to another, along with an erratic diet, was producing enough stress to keep her GI symptoms in full force.

When Sara came to us, she said she knew she should probably change her diet, but she didn't know what to change. It seemed that no matter what she ate, she got sick. We started Sara on the Two-Week Master Program. Even though the program is naturally high in fiber, which has been shown to be effective against IBS, we added some supplemental Metamucil, which is a natural fiber. After years of suffering, Sara saw a marked improvement in her symptoms in one week. Her swings from diarrhea to constipation straightened out, and the episodes of cramps became fewer and milder.

It's unlikely that we will understand the true cause of IBS any time soon. We know that some people seek medical help for IBS while others live with their symptoms. Researchers have tried to make something of this, distinguishing between psychological patterns of patients and nonpatients and attributing the disease to those patterns. But this has led us no closer to the answer. Why mostly young women? If stress is experienced at work, what kind of stress? If muscles contract irregularly in the bowel, is it caused by a genetic factor? If a biochemical factor is involved, what kind is it?

For the time being, we can at least relieve the symptoms. The Self-Help Nutritional Program is designed to help people suffering from both functional and organic digestive disorders. In many cases, particularly for a functional problem like IBS, the nutritional program alone is enough to completely eliminate symptoms. When serious underlying disease is present, the nutritional program can be a useful adjunct to drug therapy, often permitting lower drug doses and helping to speed recovery and prevent recurrence.

Part Two

Gastrointestinal Problems—
and How to Alleviate Them

5 Gastroesophageal Reflux
(Heartburn, Hiatal Hernia, Barrett's Esophagus)

Heartburn

Heartburn, a burning sensation or feeling of fullness in the middle of the chest, usually occurs within an hour after eating, and is often brought on by certain types of food. About 36 percent of all Americans suffer heartburn at least once a month, and about 7 percent experience it daily. For some people heartburn is so severe that it becomes incapacitating. Most heartburn sufferers feel it right underneath the breastbone, but occasionally a "referred" burning is felt in the back between the shoulder blades or in the jaw and teeth.

Why are some people bothered by heartburn while others are not? Chronic heartburn is a symptom of a disorder called reflux esophagitis, or GERD (gastroesophageal reflux disease). The cause of the disorder is a small one-way valve, called the lower esophageal sphincter (LES), located between the esophagus and the stomach. When functioning properly, the LES allows food and water to pass into the stomach, but prevents backward flow. If the LES is loose or weak, ferocious stomach acids can back up into the esophagus, causing a powerful burning sensation as the acid comes in contact with the sensitive lining of the esophagus.

Certain foods are known to weaken or "relax" the valve, making reflux more likely. A weak LES over time is enough to cause chronic heartburn. Sometimes the condition is complicated by a hiatal hernia, an oversized opening in the diaphragm that allows the stomach to protrude into the chest cavity, making reflux of acid easier. There is only a loose connection between hiatal hernia and heartburn, however. Many people with hiatal hernia have no symptoms from it.

Excessive pressure on the abdomen can also make it easier for the stomach acids to flow back into the esophagus. As a rule, anything that increases the pressure on the abdomen—obesity, straining, or tight-fitting garments—can promote backflow of stomach contents to the esophagus. For this reason, heartburn is especially common dur-

Drugs That Can Cause Heartburn

Drug	Disease Treated	Relaxes LES	Stimulates Acid
dicyclomine	spastic colon	X	
aminophylline	asthma	X	X
propranolol	hypertension; angina	X	
diltiazem; verapamil	hypertension; angina	X	
isosorbide	angina	X	

ing pregnancy. And some people experience heartburn only when their weight passes a particular limit.

Certain drugs may also contribute to heartburn by relaxing the LES or stimulating acid secretion by the stomach (see box).

For most sufferers of heartburn the burning sensation is the only problem. For a few people, however, heartburn leads to serious complications. Repeated exposure to acid can inflame the lining of the esophagus, making it so sensitive that sometimes swallowing is painful. The irritated lining may start to bleed, or an ulcer may develop in the esophagus. Bleeding may cause the person to vomit fresh bright red blood or old "coffee-ground" blood. Sometimes the bleeding goes unnoticed until the individual passes black, tarry bowel movements, indicating the presence of blood. Or blood may show up when the stool is tested by a physician.

Continuous inflammation over a long period of time may cause scar tissue to build up in the esophagus, narrowing the opening. Such a stricture makes it difficult to swallow solid food, and the esophagus will have to be dilated by a special nonsurgical procedure. Strictures are sometimes malignant, particularly for smokers and heavy alcohol users.

So, even if you think you can live with the discomfort of daily heartburn, it's important for your future health to try to bring symptoms under control. Fortunately, reflux esophagitis is rarely associated with cancer of the esophagus. Cancer of the esophagus is usually caused by smoking and alcohol (see Barrett's esophagus, below).

• Diagnosis

There is no relationship between reflux esophagitis and heart disease, although sometimes the symptoms seem similar. Because part of the esophagus is located just behind the heart, heartburn can be confused with angina, chest pain caused by inadequate blood flow to the heart. There are certain distinct differences in symptoms, however.

Heartburn is made worse by lying down and by eating fatty foods and chocolate; on the other hand, it is made better by antacids. None of these things is true for angina. Angina is usually brought on by exercise and is not helped by antacids. Even so, it is not always easy to distinguish between the two problems, and anyone experiencing chest pains should see a physician for correct diagnosis.

These symptoms are usually enough to diagnose heartburn. However, many doctors will want the suspected diagnosis confirmed by an upper GI series (barium swallow). A hiatal hernia can also be seen on this type of x-ray. A barium swallow is always ordered when an individual has difficulty or pain in swallowing.

To distinguish heartburn from angina, a Bernstein test is given. A pH probe and EKG may also be used.

• Treatment

Heartburn responds extremely well to the dietary guidelines established by the Self-Help Nutritional Program. Nutrition, along with some valuable changes in lifestyle, is the best treatment for heartburn. The program helps neutralize stomach acids. It is also naturally low in fat, a major culprit behind heartburn. High-fat foods are retained in the stomach longer and also tend to relax the LES valve between the esophagus and the stomach, which makes it easier for acid to back up. For more tips on preventing heartburn, see Chapter 24.

If you have a sudden attack of heartburn, sit up or stand up. Loosen restrictive clothing such as a belt or waistband. Take a dose of a liquid antacid such as Mylanta, Maalox, or Riopan. You can start with two tablespoons and go up to six tablespoons, if needed. Don't smoke or drink alcohol or coffee.

People who suffer from frequent heartburn can make the following lifestyle changes to ease the discomfort.

Meals. Avoiding lying down for at least three hours after meals, and avoid eating for several hours before bedtime.

Sleeping Habits. Many people who suffer from heartburn sleep with a pile of pillows under their head to keep stomach acid from backing up. Sleeping on pillows is not very effective because only your head and neck are elevated while your chest and torso remain flat. Sleeping on extra pillows can also cause your body to jackknife, actually increasing pressure on the abdomen and making reflux worse.

Heartburn can be vastly relieved if you can permanently elevate the head of your bed on 6-inch blocks. Elevating the head of the bed means that your body is in a comfortable position and your whole torso is raised; to back up into the esophagus, stomach acids would have to flow uphill.

Clothing. Avoid wearing tight clothing.

Weight. If you are overweight, especially if the excess weight is around your waist, lose some weight. The Self-Help Nutritional Program will naturally keep your weight under control, but you may first need to cut calories and increase exercise to establish your ideal weight (see Part Six).

Flag Foods. Pay special attention to Flag Foods for heartburn in Chapter 24. The idea is to avoid the foods that relax the LES valve and that increase stomach acid. The big culprits are fat, alcohol, and chocolate.

Medication. A lot of heart medications such as calcium channel blockers, nitrates, and beta blockers decrease LES pressure and aggravate heartburn. If you take OTC or prescription medications for any medical problems, check with your physician to make sure they are not making your heartburn worse by inadvertently causing the LES valve to relax.

Antacids. You can further neutralize the acid in your stomach by taking a dose of liquid antacid one hour after meals, the time that most acid is being released into the stomach. Add a bedtime dose because that is when acid is most likely to make its way backward into the esophagus. In addition, you can take a dose of antacid anytime you experience heartburn.

• Advanced Measures

The measures mentioned above are all things you can do yourself to relieve the daily discomfort of heartburn. If you still experience heartburn after following the Self-Help Nutritional Program for four weeks and incorporating these recommendations, see your physician.

Several prescription medications are available to relieve severe heartburn by blocking acid secretion from the stomach (Tagamet, Zantac, Pepcid, or Axid). These so-called H_2-receptor antagonist drugs reduce heartburn by healing the esophagus. Many doctors, including myself, use this class of drug as a first-line treatment for heartburn because of its overall safety and effectiveness. Occasionally the recommended dosage of these drugs—e.g., Zantac 150 milligrams twice a day—has to be doubled, or even tripled, in order to effectively relieve symptoms. At the time of writing this book only Zantac has been approved by the Federal Drug Administration (FDA) for treatment of reflux.

Metaclopramide (trade name Reglan) is another class of drug that helps prevent acid reflux by strengthening the LES valve. It also encourages acid to empty downward into the duodenum. Reglan is often used in combination with antacids or one of the H_2-receptor antagonists. However, many people who use this drug suffer side effects such as lethargy, depression, and abnormal muscle reactions, which limit its use.

A new drug called omeprazole (Prilosec) also approved by the FDA for reflux can be used when other measures fail to control symptoms. Prilosec is the most powerful acid-inhibiting drug available. A single dose of 20 milligrams can almost totally block acid secretion for a full day. Although effective, the long-term effects of Prilosec are still unknown, and its use is limited to two months.

All drugs have a potential for side effects, and none is a substitute for an overall health program.

Rarely do all measures fail to relieve symptoms. If the heartburn is severe and disabling, you may be a candidate for surgery to increase the strength of the LES. Although this is an effective procedure, it is necessary for only a small percentage of patients these days and is performed only if medical management has proved fruitless over a long period of time.

Hiatal Hernia

The esophagus passes through an opening in the diaphragm—the muscular wall dividing the chest cavity from the abdominal cavity—known as the hiatus. When this opening becomes weakened and stretched, allowing a portion of the stomach to bulge through into the chest cavity, the condition is referred to as a hiatal hernia. This is actually a very common anomaly and often does not cause any discomfort or unusual symptoms.

In some people a hiatal hernia may contribute to a weak LES, which permits backflow of stomach acid into the esophagus, making symptoms of heartburn worse. For that reason, all of the treatments advised to relieve heartburn can also be applied when hiatal hernia produces symptoms.

Barrett's Esophagus

When heartburn goes on unabated and untreated over a long period of time, acid reflux from the stomach can cause the lining of the esophagus to change, from the usual squamous cells to glandular cells reminiscent of those in the stomach or intestinal lining. This so-called Barrett's esophagus—initiated by heartburn—can also make heartburn worse. The changed lining can secrete acid directly into the esophagus, which will frequently develop an ulcer.

The risk of cancer of the esophagus is increased in people who have Barrett's esophagus. For that reason, they require regular checkups by their physicians, and some gastroenterologists recommend screening once a year by endoscopy.

Treating Barrett's esophagus with medical or even surgical intervention will not usually reverse the changes in the lining. The best treatment for Barrett's is to prevent its development by treating even mild heartburn.

6   *Peptic Ulcer Disease*

*P*eptic ulcer disease is a group of disorders in which a portion of the mucous membrane that lines the stomach and the duodenum (the first portion of the small intestine) becomes inflamed or ulcerated. Peptic ulcer disease is so common in our society that the most profitable prescription drug sold worldwide is an ulcer drug called Zantac.

Inflammation is called gastritis when it is in the stomach, and duodenitis when it is in the duodenum.

Ulcers in either location are called peptic, named for the digestive enzyme that breaks down protein.

Inflammation

Inflammation has many causes: drugs, ingestion of corrosive substances, infection, shock, surgery or other significant physical stress, allergies, and alcohol—anything that might cause the stomach to produce excessive acid or weaken the mucous membrane that lines the stomach. Gastritis and duodenitis are not usually serious conditions, but they can sometimes cause significant bleeding. These are both usually curable conditions, but if neglected can lead to complications.

• Gastritis

Gastritis, an inflammation of the stomach lining, causes discomfort in the upper abdomen, nausea, and vomiting. Eating usually makes symptoms worse. Gastritis may come on suddenly, or it may be a chronic condition that develops gradually over several years. It is commonly caused by aspirin or alcohol. In some people extreme physical stress or the development of liver failure can cause gastritis.

Chronic gastritis may be caused by prolonged irritation of the stomach by alcohol or tobacco smoke.

Gastritis is often confused with a stomach ulcer. Correct diagnosis is made by examining the stomach lining through an endoscope, a long slender tube passed down the esophagus to the stomach. A bit of tissue can be removed through the endoscope for analysis to determine the type of inflammation.

The same drugs used to treat ulcers (see below) are used successfully to treat gastritis.

• Duodenitis

Inflammation of the duodenum produces the same vague symptoms, a burning sensation in the upper abdomen. Diagnosis of duodenitis is made by endoscopy—examining the walls of the duodenum with a fiberoptic viewing tube passed through the esophagus, stomach, and pylorus. If the condition is duodenitis, there will be a diffuse area of inflammation, with redness and swelling of the lining, but no visible ulcer.

The treatment for duodenitis is similar to treatment for a duodenal ulcer (see below).

Peptic Ulcers

A peptic ulcer is a chronic sore extending through the protective mucous membrane lining the GI tract and penetrating the underlying muscle. An ulcer can form in any area exposed to gastric acid and pepsin, the digestive enzyme that helps break down protein. An ulcer may occur in the stomach (gastric ulcer), the duodenum (duodenal ulcer), or, less commonly, in the esophagus.

The cause of peptic ulcers is unknown. Ulcers occur only in the presence of stomach acid, but they are not necessarily caused by excessive quantities of acid. Even people who produce low levels of acid sometimes develop ulcers; others who produce large amounts of acid may be ulcer-free. Distortion of the balance between acid and protective mucus is the likely cause. With inadequate "mucosal defense," even a small amount of acid can cause an ulcer.

Several factors, including stress, are known to affect the production of acid and mucus. However, some people under great stress never develop ulcers, while others who lead seemingly quiet lives do. Certain drugs—aspirin and other nonsteroidal anti-inflammatory drugs (NSAIDs)—can erode the lining. Smoking and alcohol consumption may exacerbate ulcers, but probably do not cause them. Nor do spicy foods appear to be the cause. Some people may simply be born with a sensitive stomach lining or a tendency to produce excessive acid.

Regardless of the cause, ulcer pain is usually worse when the stomach is empty because acid can more readily come in contact with the irritated lining of the stomach or duodenum. Food helps set up a barrier and tends to neutralize acid.

Ulcers that occur in the stomach usually cause pain in the upper middle of your abdomen (epigastrium), or just below your rib cage on the left side. Eating may aggravate stomach ulcers at first, especially certain foods, but then the burning sensation subsides as the food begins to buffer the stomach acid. Stomach ulcers occur more often in people over the age of forty. This higher incidence in older people may be caused by increased use of drugs such as aspirin and NSAIDs which are often used to treat arthritis. (See Part Three for information about NSAID-induced ulcers.)

Duodenal ulcers usually occur in younger people between the ages of twenty and forty, probably because younger people produce more acid. Burning pain from duodenal ulcers may be felt in the epigastrium or a little to the right. Eating often relieves the pain quickly because of an immediate buffering effect, but irritants in certain foods can produce more pain.

Men tend to have a higher incidence of all kinds of ulcers, although this phenomenon is changing as more women suffer the ramifications of high-stress jobs. Stress seems to stimulate the production of chemicals that in turn promote excessive stomach acid. People under stress also tend to eat erratically, drink too much, and smoke cigarettes, all of which can invite an ulcer. As of now, about 10 percent of American men will develop some form of ulcers in their lifetime.

• Ulcer Treatment

Drug therapy is always recommended to treat ulcers because drugs help speed healing. Untreated, ulcers can bleed, perforate, or cause obstruction, and it is best to heal them as quickly as possible. Ulcers are seldom malignant, although any gastric ulcer is potentially malignant and needs to be evaluated, especially if you are over forty years old. Three types of drugs are used to heal ulcers: antacids to neutralize the stomach acid; H_2-receptor antagonists to inhibit acid production; and sucralfate to protectively coat the ulcer.

Antacids neutralize excess acidity: one tablet or one tablespoon of an antacid such as Maalox or Mylanta is given one and three hours after meals, at bedtime, and as needed to control symptoms. (Studies show that low doses of antacids work just as well as larger doses.) Antacid therapy properly used may be as effective as other prescription drugs (see below). For many people, antacids taken regularly can ultimately relieve pain and, along with changes in diet and lifestyle, may be enough to heal the ulcer.

Many physicians prefer to use the H_2-receptor antagonists (Tagamet, Zantac, Pepcid, Axid) as the first line of treatment. These drugs are considered by many to be the gold standard for treating peptic ulcer disease.

This class of drug works by inhibiting acid secretion in the stomach. Acid is secreted by specialized gastric cells in the stomach, which are stimulated by a chemical called histamine. H_2-receptor antagonists are structurally similar to histamine, and they stick to the acid-producing cells the way a key fits into a lock, blocking the real histamine from reaching the cell. A standard dose of H_2 blocker can knock out acid production by about 70 percent.

Another new acid inhibitor, recently approved by the FDA for reflux, is Prilosec (omeprazole). Prilosec inhibits acid secretion by blocking hydrogen-potassium ATPase, the enzyme responsible for expelling acid from the gastric cell. The drug is so effective it can eliminate acid secretion for hours and even days at a time. However, some safety issues are still unresolved. Because Prilosec inhibits acid secretion so profoundly it causes release of a hormone called gastrin, which in turn stimulates growth of certain stomach cells. Studies in rats that received Prilosec for over two years (basically the lifetime of a rat) showed that long-standing levels of gastrin in the stomach produced malignant tumors in the stomach. To date, there is no evidence that Prilosec causes similar tumors in humans.

Another type of drug, sucralfate or Carafate, works by binding to the raw exposed surface of inflamed or ulcerated tissue and forming a protective coat, which allows healing to occur. These drugs, only weak suppressors of acid secretion, nevertheless work as well as antacids or H_2 blockers.

• Recurrent Ulcer Disease

The recurrence rate for ulcers is high. Once an ulcer is healed, you have a 75 percent chance of developing another one within a year's time. Recurrence can usually be prevented by using a half-dose of an H_2-receptor antagonist as maintenance to reduce acid production (e.g., Zantac 150 mg at bedtime, Pepcid 20 mg at bedtime, etc.). This kind of preventive therapy is about 75-percent effective. The problem is that as soon as the maintenance dose is stopped, your risk of recurrence resumes. For this reason, some physicians do not put their patients on maintenance doses, preferring to take a wait-and-see approach. Drug therapy is begun again only if the ulcer recurs.

New evidence suggests that peptic ulcer disease is an infectious disease caused by a bacterium called *Helicobacter pylori*. Every person with duodenal ulcers has this bacterium present in the stomach, but only about 40 percent of people without ulcers have it, and only 40 to 50 percent of people with gastric ulcers have it. The bacterium is thought to be responsible for relapses of duodenal ulcer disease.

Specific recommendations have not yet been clearly formulated for the treatment of *Helicobacter pylori*. Antibiotics frequently cause nausea and diarrhea and are not always effective against this stubborn bacterium; for these reasons, they are seldom used initially to treat ulcers, even if the organism is found on a biopsy of the stomach antrum (the last portion of· the stomach that empties into the duodenum). Antibiotic treatment is usually reserved for the rare patient who does not respond to conventional therapy or for those who have frequent recurrences.

Many gastroenterologists, myself included, combine antibiotics with Pepto-Bismol for these patients. The major active ingredient in Pepto-Bismol is bismuth subsalicylate, which appears to suppress the growth of bacteria, particularly *Helicobacter pylori*.

Self-Help

The Self-Help Nutritional Program, in conjunction with drug therapy, can help relieve the symptoms of peptic ulcer disease. After the condition is healed, the Self-Help Nutritional Program, which is high in fiber, may help reduce the incidence of recurrence. This can be important for patients who do not take maintenance drug therapy. However, dietary therapy cannot be relied on to prevent ulcer recurrence.

One patient of mine with peptic ulcer disease demonstrates how it often takes a combination of drug therapy, along with changes in lifestyle and diet, to heal and manage ulcers. Brendan, a thirty-five-year-old rising star in his management consulting firm, began his day with an hour of paper work on a commuter train, and ended it the same way, twelve hours later. His normal breakfast consisted of four cups of strong coffee, three cigarettes, and a danish. He made time for lunch only when entertaining a client.

On the way home from work at night, Brendan usually nursed a Scotch on the rocks and smoked five more cigarettes. Around 8:30 p.m.

he would eat a huge meal when, he said, he could finally relax and enjoy food. The foods he enjoyed most were curries, red-hot Italian tomato sauces, and any Mexican food as long as it had plenty of salsa.

For the last two months Brendan had awakened with a burning, gnawing sensation in the pit of his stomach and a feeling of nausea. Eating a cracker usually helped subdue the gnawing feeling. His wife joked that he might be pregnant. His symptoms tended to return in the late afternoon. One day he noticed a dark tarry bowel movement. Brendan called his family physician, who referred him to me.

His physical exam was normal, except for mild tenderness when I pressed on the epigastric area. A complete blood count was within the normal range so it was unlikely that Brendan had lost a lot of blood, and there was no evidence of active bleeding.

I concluded that it was safe to send him home. I ordered an upper GI series and, as a preliminary treatment before making a definite diagnosis, prescribed an H_2 blocker that he could take once a day—which I thought was more in keeping with his lifestyle than multiple-dose drugs. I also told him to carry antacid tablets in his pocket in case his symptoms became suddenly uncomfortable during the day or night.

We discussed the stresses in his life and "taking time to smell the roses," but this advice was largely lost on Brendan. He wasn't interested in changing his charged-up lifestyle. However, he listened to advice about dietary management. I recommended cutting back on coffee and using decaf, if possible. I also prescribed a quick high-fiber cereal for breakfast, a sandwich and decaf beverage for lunch, and eliminating alcohol and spices from his diet. I told him the importance of three meals a day in order to avoid long periods of fasting.

I reminded him that since he is allowed to smoke neither at home or at work (thank goodness for take-charge wives, obnoxious non-smokers, and the Clean Air Bill), he might as well give up smoking altogether. He said he would try, but didn't sound as if he meant it.

One week later he returned feeling much better. His symptoms had disappeared. The upper GI series showed that Brendan had a small ulcer crater in the duodenal bulb, confirming my diagnosis of peptic ulcer disease. I told him to continue the H_2 blocker for a total of eight weeks and to call if his symptoms returned. I gave him a home test to check his stool for blood. He was still smoking.

Nonulcer Dyspepsia

At least half of people who have ulcerlike pain—a gnawing or burning discomfort in the pit of the stomach—do not have anything visibly wrong with the lining of their stomach or duodenum when the GI tract is examined endoscopically. This symptom complex is called nonulcer dyspepsia. It is often localized to one area, occurs most often early in the morning, and is often relieved by antacids and food. Dyspepsia may not respond to conventional antiulcer drugs, and the best treatment is self-help measures.

Food. Avoid spicy sauces, coffee, tea, cola, alcoholic beverages, orange juice, tomato juice, and radishes.

Drugs. Antacids may be taken one hour after each meal and at bedtime, or even every hour to relieve pain. *Do not* take aspirin or aspirin-containing products, ibuprofen, or other anti-inflammatory medicines to relieve stomach pain. Stop smoking.

If the pain is severe, or if it persists or recurs, see your physician. Stomach pain may be caused by gallbladder attacks, inflammation of the pancreas, or ulcers. In older adults, there's even a small chance that such pain could be caused by stomach cancer. So if you experience stomach pain repeatedly, it's important to get a proper diagnosis by your physician.

7 *Pancreatitis*

*B*urning pain in the upper abdomen can also be caused by an inflamed pancreas, the oblong organ that lies within the curvature of the duodenum and extends toward the spleen, which puts it in close proximity to several vital structures.

The pancreas is divided into two independent sections: the endocrine section secretes many important hormones, including insulin, directly into the bloodstream; the exocrine section produces a wide variety of digestive enzymes that process food into a form that can be absorbed by the small intestine. The exocrine section also secretes a bicarbonate-rich fluid that is important in neutralizing stomach acids. Pancreatitis affects primarily the exocrine pancreas.

Pancreatitis may be acute or chronic. In acute pancreatitis the gland usually returns to normal after a single attack. In chronic pancreatitis there is permanent damage to the gland and its function is impaired.

Acute Pancreatitis

• Symptoms and Causes

The most important symptom of acute pancreatitis is steady stomach pain in the upper abdomen (epigastrium), sometimes spreading to the back. The pain is usually severe, although sometimes it is quite mild or diffuse. The pain is usually worse when you move around or lie down, but eases when you sit up and lean forward.

On ultrasound or CAT scan the pancreas may appear enlarged, but an accurate diagnosis of acute pancreatitis is usually confirmed by laboratory tests that measure a rise in serum amylase, a pancreatic enzyme released into the blood during an attack.

The principal cause of acute pancreatitis in men is alcohol abuse; in women it is gallstones. Other less common causes include an ulcer on the portion of the duodenum next to the pancreas, injury (such as surgery on the biliary tract or a blow to the abdomen), high levels of calcium or triglycerides in the blood, and certain drugs (sulfa drugs, thiazide diuretics, steroids, and birth control pills).

• Treatment

Acute pancreatitis usually requires hospitalization and intravenous fluids. It may be associated with vomiting, fever, severe abdominal pain, and shock. No solid food can be taken during an acute episode. Unfortunately, drugs do not help. If gallstones or another obstruction is the cause of an acute episode, they can be removed surgically or, sometimes, through the endoscope.

It may take several days, or even several weeks, for an acute episode to pass and for the pancreas to return to normal functioning. Some scarring may remain. If the cause of the attack is removed—if the gallstones are removed or, if alcohol was the precipitating factor, if the individual stops drinking—a recurrence is unlikely.

Chronic Pancreatitis

• Symptoms and Causes

Chronic pancreatitis is a progressive disease that over a period of months and years slowly destroys the cells of the exocrine pancreas. Symptoms may be the same as in the acute form, with attacks becoming more frequent as they continue. Rarely, there may be no pain at all. The principal signs of the disease may be weight loss and elevated blood sugars.

Chronic pancreatitis seems to result from a cascade of events, often beginning with alcohol abuse. Sometimes repeated acute episodes lead to a chronic condition, especially if alcohol abuse is involved.

As chronic pancreatitis progresses, the endocrine pancreas may also be destroyed, and diabetes is the result. Digestion continues normally until about 90 percent of enzyme production is destroyed. When production finally shuts down, food can no longer be processed and therefore cannot be absorbed by the small intestine.

People with chronic pancreatitis may lose weight and have large bulky stools. They may be ravenously hungry, often consuming enough extra food to maintain body weight. The extra food intake often puts a strain on the damaged pancreas and causes pain. Some people with severe pain cannot compensate for their inefficient digestion by eating more food and will lose a significant amount of weight.

Measuring pancreatic enzymes in the blood is of no use in making the diagnosis because serum amylase levels usually are not elevated in the chronic form of pancreatitis. Abdominal x-rays or scans may be ordered, along with a special endoscopic procedure called endoscopic retrograde cholangiopancreatography (ERCP), which allows the physician to view the extent of tissue damage.

• Treatment

Blood sugar levels can be controlled by giving insulin. Pancreatic extract can be given to correct the underproduction of enzymes caused by the condition. Pain management is a critical part of the treatment picture. At this time, except for addicting painkillers, no drugs can help the pain of chronic pancreatitis. Certain drugs that block pancreatic secretion (e.g., high doses of pancreatic extract) may help rest the pancreas and thus provide some relief, but often this therapy is not sufficient to control pain, especially in alcoholics.

New drugs are in development that may be effective in treating the pain of chronic pancreatitis. Sandostatin (octreotide acetate), a synthetic hormone that inhibits pancreatic secretion, is currently marketed for treatment of severe diarrhea, but some studies suggest that it may also help in both acute and chronic pancreatitis.

Cholecystokinin (CCK), a hormone released from the intestines into the bloodstream by digestion of dietary fat or protein, is the major stimulant to the pancreas after a meal. Drugs are being developed to block CCK and thus prevent pancreatic secretion. Unfortunately, CCK also stimulates gallbladder function; if CCK is blocked, the gallbladder will be unable to empty bile, which could lead to the development of gallstones.

Because management of the pain of chronic pancreatitis has been so unrewarding, patients with persistent pain are often treated surgically—either by removing most of the pancreas or, if possible, draining the pancreatic duct. Even with surgery, only about three-fourths of patients experience a reduction of pain. Obviously, before resorting to surgery, every effort should be made to control pancreatitis with dietary management and drug therapy, while at the same time avoiding narcotics.

Self-Help

Gabriel, a forty-two-year-old computer salesman, had a burning pain in the pit of his stomach that felt as if it was boring straight through to his back. The pain was unremitting. It became worse when he ate and seemed unbearable whenever he lay down. He tried antacids, which did not help. His family physician ordered an upper GI series, but nothing showed up. An ultrasound of his gallbladder showed no evidence of gallstones. Blood tests were normal, although on one occasion serum amylase was slightly elevated.

When Gabriel was referred to me, we talked about his life. He told me that he had separated from his wife three years before. He had always entertained clients with three-martini lunches, but over the last few years his alcohol consumption had gradually increased. He now drank a fifth of vodka a day and had several glasses of wine with meals. His sales performance had worsened and he had received a few warnings from his boss regarding his working hours and sales quota.

I felt Gabriel had the classic signs and symptoms of chronic pancreatitis. I performed endoscopic retrograde cholangiopancreatography (ERCP) on Gabriel, passing a flexible tube with a light down his esophagus, through the stomach, and into the duodenum, to locate the openings of the pancreatic duct. (The tube is similar to an endoscope except the light and optics are on the side, rather than the tip.) Dye was then injected to fill the duct, and x-ray pictures were taken to show any abnormalities. In this case, the x-rays revealed a dilated duct with several narrowed areas.

The immediate treatment for Gabriel was to get him off alcohol to stop further destruction of his pancreas. I arranged for a three-week inpatient detoxification and a referral to Alcoholics Anonymous. At the same time, I started him on a low-fat, high-carbohydrate diet, identical to the Two-Week Master Program. The pain that usually occurred when he ate was reduced. We added high doses of pancreatic extract, and that further reduced pain. Although he was not completely pain-free, he was able to get by without narcotics and without surgery.

If you asked Gabriel what helped him the most, he would tell you that the low-fat diet brought the greatest pain relief. The Self-Help Nutritional Program is enormously helpful in managing chronic pancreatitis because it helps reduce stimulation of the pancreas. Smaller meals throughout the day may produce less pain than larger meals. People suffering from pancreatic failure can also get some additional nutritional help by taking prescription pancreatic extracts to replace digestive enzymes. Alcohol should be strictly avoided.

8   *Gallbladder Problems*

The gallbladder is a pear-shaped sac with thin, smooth walls lying just underneath the liver and attached to it by fibrous tissue. The liver produces quantities of yellowish-green bile; a system of bile ducts carries the bile from the liver into the gallbladder where it is stored. When you eat fatty foods, the gallbladder contracts and pushes the bile back through the ducts into the small intestine where it helps digest the fat. Normally the gallbladder and bile duct do their vital work unnoticed. Sometimes, however, the gallbladder malfunctions. When a fatty meal makes a diseased gallbladder contract, the result can be a chronic nagging "grungy" feeling in the right upper quadrant of the abdomen. This is a very common condition.

Cholecystitis (inflammation of the gallbladder) is a common disorder of the gallbladder and is usually caused by the formation of gallstones. (Gallbladder inflammation without stones present, called acalculous cholcystitis, may be brought on by prolonged fasting, severe illness, or no obvious reason at all.)

Although more than 20 million Americans have gallstones, the stones do not always cause problems. About 80 percent of people who have them never notice them at all; even if the stones are discovered by a physician they will be left untreated unless they begin to cause symptoms.

Gallstone Types and Symptoms

There are three main types of gallstones: cholesterol stones, pigmented stones, and mixed stones. In America, most gallstones are cholesterol or mixed gallstones, and women are affected four times as often as men. (In Asia, gallstones are more often pigmented.)

If a gallstone becomes lodged in the neck of the gallbladder or stuck in the duct it may irritate and inflame the gallbladder walls and can be the source of considerable pain. The most common symptom is a sharp pain or a painful spasm on the right side, just under the rib cage. Sometimes you can feel the pain radiate to your back under the right shoulder blade. Symptoms often flare after meals because the gallbladder normally contracts after you eat fatty or greasy foods.

Treatment

On three separate occasions, Bernadette experienced severe pain on her right side, just under the rib cage, about three hours after eating fatty food. Once the pain was so severe that it traveled to her back and she vomited green bile. Bernadette had all the risk factors for gallstones: she was a woman, she was over age forty, and she was overweight. Ultrasound confirmed that she had a solitary stone measuring 1.5 centimeters or ⅝ of an inch across.

We attempted to dissolve the stone without surgery (see below), and recommended a low-fat diet similar to the Two-Week Master Program. Bernadette did well on the diet and her symptoms completely disappeared—until one afternoon when she indulged in a couple of slices of pizza. She immediately experienced pain on her right side. This convinced her of the importance of diet therapy.

The Self-Help Nutritional Program is ideal for people with gallbladder problems of all kinds because it is naturally low in fats, which means that fewer demands are placed on the gallbladder and it contracts less forcefully. Therefore, although the program cannot actually dissolve gallstones, it may reduce the frequency and severity of painful attacks. Because dietary fiber reduces the amount of cholesterol in bile, the tendency to form gallstones is also reduced. By changing the chemical composition of the bile through diet, it is possible to halt the growth of stones or in rare cases, even cause the stones to shrink.

In the past, all troublesome gallstones were treated by surgically removing the gallbladder. Although surgery still remains an important treatment option, gallstones can sometimes be dissolved medically, leaving the gallbladder intact. At the Comprehensive Gallstone Treatment Center at Thomas Jefferson University Hospital, patients who have three or fewer small, uncalcified stones and a functioning gallbladder can undergo a treatment called *extracorporeal shockwave lithotripsy*. In this treatment the individual is sedated while lying on a special table that submerges the right upper abdomen in a water bath, which conducts the shockwaves. The stones are located by ultrasound, and their exact location is fed into a computer, which automatically aims the shockwaves at the stones. This causes the stones to vibrate and ultimately shatter into tiny particles of gravel. A single shockwave treatment is followed by several months of drug therapy with ursodiol

(Actigall), a bile salt, which fully dissolves the gravel. Actigall can be used without lithotripsy if a patient has multiple small gallstones and the gallbladder is functioning.

The Self-Help Nutritional Program can be an important part of gallstone treatment. While the individual is on medication, a forceful contraction of the gallbladder after fat ingestion can cause small fragments of gravel to travel into the bile duct where they can become trapped, blocking the duct and causing the bile to back up into the bloodstream. The resulting symptoms include a yellow tinge to the skin (yellow jaundice), pain in the upper right abdomen (biliary colic), and fever due to infection in the bile ducts (cholangitis). The Two-Week Master Program is low in fat, making forceful contraction of the gallbladder less likely.

Obesity, Dieting, and Gallstones

Recently there has been controversy over whether dieting to lose weight causes gallstones. It is well known that obesity itself causes cholesterol gallstones to form. In fact the heavier you are, the greater your risk for gallstones. An adult of normal weight without symptoms of gallbladder disease has about a 9 percent risk of having gallstones. That risk increases twofold for mild obesity (20 to 30 percent above ideal body weight) and up to sixfold for morbid obesity (more than 100 percent above ideal body weight).

Some studies suggest that the risk of developing gallstones may increase transiently during active weight loss. These studies were all done using either stomach bypass surgery or very-low-calorie diets (about 500 calories a day). In the studies using very-low-calorie diets, ultrasound of the gallbladder was performed before and after losing weight. About 25 percent of obese subjects who did not have gallstones detectable by ultrasound before dieting had detectable stones after losing weight.

One of the major problems of the studies is that it is difficult to detect gallstones by ultrasound in obese subjects. The stones found after significant weight loss may just have been gallstones missed on the initial study.

If very-low-calorie diets do on occasion cause gallstones, it may be related to poor stimulation of the gallbladder—with less fat (1–2 grams a day) there is less gallbladder contraction. Stagnant bile loaded with cholesterol is the setting for gallstone formation.

At this time, there is no evidence that diets of higher calorie and fat value (750 calories or above) cause gallstones. However, high calorie intake (greater than 3000 calories per day) or high cholesterol intake (greater than 1000 milligrams of cholesterol per day) are associated with gallstone formation.

The good news is that after you have lost your excess weight, your risk of developing gallstones goes back to normal. Considering the health risks of remaining obese (such as heart disease, diabetes, cancer, stroke, and infertility), I feel it is imperative to try to lose weight with an appropriate combination of diet and exercise (see Chapters 27 and 28).

9   *Irritable Bowel Syndrome (IBS)*

*I*rritable bowel syndrome (IBS) is really a constella-
tion of symptoms, usually involving a change in bowel habits, abdominal pain, and excessive gas. A person with IBS may have a single
symptom or a combination of several of these problems.

IBS is one of the most common health problems in the Western
hemisphere. For some reason, young women tend to be much more
susceptible to IBS than men. IBS is sometimes called colitis, but in
fact this is a misnomer because no "itis," or inflammation, is present.
It also goes by the names of spastic colon, spastic colitis, and mucous
colitis. All of this nomenclature means the same thing—irritable
bowel syndrome.

Symptoms of IBS

Many healthy people commonly have gastrointestinal complaints
several times a year, including abdominal pain, constipation, and
diarrhea. If they decide to visit a physician for a diagnosis—which
most do not—the symptoms may be confused with those of serious
structural abnormalities, such as inflammation of the bowel (colitis)
or cancer. In IBS no such structural abnormality exists. In fact, the
diagnosis depends on having normal results from diagnostic tests,
including a barium enema, sigmoidoscopy, an upper GI series and
small bowel follow-through, stool culture, and analysis for white cells
and parasites.

When all of these test results are normal but symptoms persist,
the condition is defined as IBS. Make no mistake, this is a real physiological disorder, not a psychosomatic ailment as was originally
thought. IBS means that the bowel does not contract properly. It may
contract forcefully after eating, causing severe cramps or spasm. Diarrhea may occur from hypermotility of the bowel. Or normal contractions of the bowel may *decrease* in frequency or become weaker,

leading to constipation. Sometimes constipation occurs because slower transit through the colon allows more time for fluid to be absorbed from the stool. The common symptoms of IBS, then, are painful spasms and bloating, usually in the lower abdomen, and diarrhea or constipation—very commonly, diarrhea alternating with constipation. Sometimes mucus is produced in excess and may be seen coating the surface of the stool.

Many people with IBS notice that their abdominal pain subsides after a bowel movement. By contrast, pain tends to increase when more frequent loose bowel movements occur. Some people feel they have had an incomplete bowel movement and need to go again. While this symptom, called tenesmus, is associated with IBS, it can also occur when there is a tumor on the colon. For this reason, anyone who has tenesmus as a symptom should have a workup that includes sigmoidoscopy and a barium enema or colonoscopy to rule out the possibility of a more serious ailment.

It's interesting that even when IBS symptoms are severe they rarely disturb a person's sleep. If symptoms do arise in the night, it usually suggests that some organic problem, such as inflammatory bowel disease or long-standing diabetes, is the cause.

IBS may be present from infancy, but tends to begin in young adulthood. A young person with only IBS symptoms and no other manifestation of organic disease—no fever, rectal bleeding, or weight loss—usually doesn't require diagnostic studies. Adults past the age of forty or fifty who begin to suffer from IBS symptoms can usually recall having had similar episodes in the past. Even so, when an older person begins to have these symptoms, they should be evaluated with a full diagnostic workup to rule out potentially serious GI disease.

Treatment

Melissa was a twenty-three-year-old secretary who complained of abdominal cramps. She had had this problem since her early teens. It would become especially severe before exams and during dates in high school. The pain was in the left and right lower abdomen. It was worse just before moving her bowels, and improved after a bowel movement.

Melissa also had frequent episodes of diarrhea, containing mucus but no visible blood. Then she would go for days without moving her bowels. Her symptoms of diarrhea seemed to get worse around the time of her period. She had recently seen her gynecologist for a pelvic exam, which proved to be normal. Because Melissa is sexually active the gynecologist cultured her cervix for mycoplasma and gonococcus. Both tests were negative.

Melissa had none of the symptoms more characteristic of inflammatory bowel disease (rectal bleeding, fever). But at times her symptoms were so severe she would hunch over and clutch her abdomen, and then have to run to the bathroom. Since most of her symptoms occurred during working hours, especially when she was under specific deadlines set by her unsympathetic boss, Melissa spent a good part of the day in the ladies' room.

Except for the usual childhood diseases, Melissa had no past history of illness. She did not smoke cigarettes and had stopped drinking alcohol because it "gave her the runs." No one in her family had ever had colon cancer or inflammatory bowel disease.

Melissa's physical examination was entirely within normal limits except for some mild discomfort in the lower abdomen. I felt she had the classic symptoms of IBS and did not warrant any further diagnostic evaluation. That was the good news. The bad news was that although IBS is not considered a serious medical disorder, it is usually impossible to control all of the symptoms all of the time.

IBS may stay the same or worsen over time; it is usually an intermittent, lifelong condition that may require lifetime management. One of the important goals of treatment is to instill a positive attitude. For that reason, I believe it's important to avoid negative labels when speaking of IBS. I use the word "condition" or "disorder" to describe IBS rather than the word "disease," even though according to the strict definition of disease as "a condition of the living animal or plant body or one of its parts that impairs the performance of a vital function," IBS is a disease. Further, even though there are no structural abnormalities in IBS patients, there are some well-defined abnormalities in the motility, or movement, of the colon.

Reassurance that symptoms are not serious goes a long way in helping individuals deal with IBS: there are no strict rules about what is a normal bowel movement, and some abdominal discomfort associated with colonic spasms is normal for some people. It also comforts my female patients to know that so many of them have IBS, so they are not alone. Since some of the symptoms of IBS are personal, women tend not to tell their friends about it. One of my patients came back to see me after taking a quick poll of her friends, family, and fellow office workers: 30 percent suffered from IBS symptoms.

On the other hand, I have found that once people start talking about their bowels they may go on and on with whoever will politely listen. I try to discourage this type of obsessive talking in order to encourage taking one's mind off the disorder and getting on with a productive life. I once told Mrs. Frawley, an elderly patient of mine, that I have a great interest in hearing about all of her bowel complaints, but that her neighbors and Mr. Frawley (who had called me the week before) would prefer that she and I dealt with this problem alone. The result was that my visit with her now lasts one hour instead of thirty minutes, and she still seeks "outside help" with her delicate complaints.

I am not a therapeutic nihilist when it comes to IBS treatment. At times, antispasmodic drugs can alleviate the painful lower abdominal cramps (see Part Three). Fiber products, stool softeners, and laxatives can help treat constipation; fiber products, antispasmodics, and other antidiarrheal products can help treat diarrhea. However, as with any kind of medical therapy, you have to consider the cost-and-risk-to-benefit ratios. Many of the drugs used to treat IBS have side effects. For example, antispasmodics such as Bentyl (dicyclomine hydrochloride and Pro-Banthine (propantheline bromide) can cause sedation, dry mouth, difficulty urinating, and a fast heart rate. Harsh laxatives can lead over time to a flaccid colon that doesn't function properly.

In addition to their potential side effects, many of these drugs are expensive and are usually only modestly effective over the long term. The long term is the real issue. IBS is a lifelong condition and by nature is relatively benign. It is difficult to recommend using strong drugs on a regular basis. However, symptoms can come on quite suddenly at times and can be severe. At times like these, intermittent drug therapy may be the best help.

By far the best approach for the long-term management of IBS symptoms is diet. A high-fiber diet significantly affects the colon, or large intestine, throughout its entire course. Fiber, with a little help from friendly bacteria residing in the colon, supplies the cells lining the colon with their primary fuel—short-chain fatty acids. With its spongelike action of holding on to water, fiber also increases the bulk of stool and helps reabsorb excess fluid. These properties make fiber useful in treating symptoms of both constipation and diarrhea. Extra bulk moves the stool through the colon faster, which relieves constipation without producing diarrhea.

A high-fiber diet is not a cure-all for IBS, but it seems to help most patients, especially those with constipation. In some people, a high-fiber diet may make symptoms of diarrhea or bloating worse, however. Usually this does not happen if vegetables and grains naturally high in fiber are gradually introduced into the diet. But a few people with IBS continue to have such symptoms and should discontinue a high-fiber program.

Anyone who suffers from the symptoms of IBS should have a medical evaluation. Many physicians prescribe an antispasmodic agent such as Donnatal (belladonna alkaloids combined with phenobarbital) or Bentyl (dicyclomine hydrochloride) for their IBS patients to have on hand in case of sudden lower abdominal cramps. Warm compresses to the lower abdomen may also ease the discomfort of cramps. Stress management can also play an important part in reducing the frequency and intensity of symptoms. Stress plays an important role in causing acute attacks of IBS, and reducing stress can help relieve the attack. The problem is that the attack may not occur until several hours after the stress has passed. Stress has a residual action in the body, almost a reverberation. Taut muscles set up a chain reaction through the gut (see Chapter 17).

In the long run, close adherence to the Self-Help Nutritional Program can help prevent IBS attacks and minimize those that do occur. And a little tender loving care and reassurance by a physician can go a long way in helping individuals suffering from IBS deal in a positive way with their symptoms.

10 *Gastrointestinal Gas*
(Gas Pain, Belching, Flatulence, Milk Intolerance)

Gas can affect the GI tract from the stomach to the anus. Eructation, or belching, bloating and distension, cramps and flatulence (passing gas from the rectum) are familiar and common symptoms related to the presence of gas in the GI tract. The type of symptom depends on where the excess gas is located. Gas in the stomach is different from gas in the colon, or large bowel.

We don't usually think of these symptoms as pathological; however, when they occur on a frequent basis they may be caused by specific gastrointestinal disorders. Some people feel gas pains or cramps even if they don't produce large amounts of gas. People with IBS, for example, have a lower threshold for pain caused by a distended colon.

Gas in the Upper GI Tract—Eructation

Eructation, or belching, is the most common symptom of gas in the upper GI tract. The composition of belched gas is similar to that of air (mostly nitrogen), which gives us a good clue to its origin. Belching is due to large amounts of air in the stomach, usually caused by excessive swallowing of air. Swallowing air is often a nervous habit related to stress and anxiety. Gulping food also tends to cause accumulation of air in the stomach. Chewing gum, sucking on a pipe or cigar for a long time, or taking long "drags" on a cigarette can also cause excessive stomach gas. Patients with severe lung disease such as emphysema tend to swallow extra air. And some people during exercise huff and puff to such an extent that some air gets swallowed.

The fate of excess swallowed air varies according to the individual and may differ at times in the same person. When you are standing up, stomach air is always in the upper part of the stomach, near the opening of the esophagus. It is normal for the LES valve between the stomach and the esophagus to relax when you swallow; if excess air is present in the stomach, a belch should follow. If this one-way valve is weak, the path of least resistance may be for the air to reflux back up into the esophagus and pass out through the mouth, leading to chronic belching.

If the air doesn't escape by belching it can get temporarily trapped in the stomach and cause bloating and a full feeling in the upper abdomen. Some people may even get painful abdominal distension. Eventually, the air will pass into the small intestine and beyond and can add to the "gas load" normally present in the bowel.

The major treatment for upper GI tract gas is to avoid excessive air swallowing. Relaxation techniques for stress management may be helpful. Giving up gum chewing, smoking, and carbonated beverages and learning to eat and drink slowly can also reduce air swallowing.

The Self-Help Nutritional Program is useful for this condition because it avoids or minimizes foods that cause the LES valve to relax. If gas is trapped in the stomach, however, you may want to encourage belching. In that case, sucking on a peppermint candy may help relax the LES, allowing you to belch and ease gas buildup in the stomach. The same action tends to cause heartburn, though—always a trade-off!

Over-the-counter medications such as Mylicon (simethicone) help break up gas bubbles and can promote belching to relieve stomach gas pains (see Part Three). If simethicone itself, or products like Mylanta, which contain simethicone, do not work, you will probably have to ride out your attack of gas pain. Fortunately, most episodes are not severe and resolve on their own within a few minutes to a few hours. You may be able to help things along by pressing on your abdomen to help move the gas out of the stomach.

Lower Intestinal Gas—Flatulence

Although swallowed air can pass into the intestines and lead to a distended, bloated abdomen and flatulence, most flatulence is caused by gas produced in the body by bacteria.

Gas buildup in the lower GI tract usually stems from the normal bacterial fermentation of food being digested. As food is digested, intestinal bacteria produce gas. Different foods produce different gases, and individuals have varying responses. Most plant foods produce methane gas. About 30 percent of the population naturally produce excessive amounts of this gas. Flatulence produced from methane gas is noticeable but fairly innocuous since methane itself is odorless.

Certain plant foods—cabbage, broccoli, brussels sprouts, cauliflower, dried apricots, and beans—are sulfurous and can produce gas that has a fairly potent odor. Beans and other legumes are major gas producers because they contain a special type of carbohydrate that is poorly absorbed but quickly digested by bacteria in your intestines.

Fiber can also cause problems. Some otherwise indigestible fiber is quite digestible by certain strains of intestinal bacteria, leading to flatulence. Milk also creates gas in many people. Lacking the enzyme to digest the lactose in milk, their intestinal bacteria have a field day and produce distension and flatus in abundance. For people who can fully digest milk, milk may cause no flatus at all. (See below.)

Everyone passes gas every day of their lives, but when it gets out of control there are several things that may help.

The high-fiber Self-Help Nutritional Program, which recommends that you *slowly incorporate fiber into your diet*, decreases flatulence by moving newly made feces rapidly through the large intestine. When some people get enthusiastic about the Self-Help Nutritional Program they suddenly increase their fiber intake from their customary 10 grams daily to 50 grams or more. The bacteria in their intestines run amok, often creating diarrhea and embarrassing quantities of gas. The amount of fiber in the recipes in this book—between 20 and 30 grams a day—should not be a major problem for most people.

By carefully checking their Flag Foods (see Chapter 24) and making some recorded observations, most people can determine which foods are most likely to produce excessive flatus for them. If you find that you still have excessive flatulence there are several antiflatus products available over the counter, but for most people these are unnecessary.

Some people don't want to eliminate gas-forming foods from their diet, and some people continue to pass gas no matter what they eat. Their primary concern is the noise and the odor. You can't eliminate the noise, but if odor is a problem for you, try two activated charcoal capsules after meals. Because activated charcoal is an absorbent, it can reduce the volume of intestinal gas by about 75 percent and deodorize the gas as well. People who have had a colostomy can also use charcoal capsules to reduce odor.

Activated charcoal is a natural product. It has enormous internal surface area, which makes it very absorbent and adsorbent, meaning that it attracts other particles to its surface. For this reason, take it at least two hours before or one hour after any medication or hormones that you might be taking for other reasons. Charcoal tablets or capsules are available without prescription at pharmacies and health food stores.

As far as drug therapy is concerned, Mylicon (simethicone) may help, although it often isn't as effective for flatulence as it is for belching.

Lactose (Milk) Intolerance

One common and little recognized cause of gas or flatulence is lactose intolerance, or lactase deficiency. *Lactase* is an enzyme produced in the intestine to digest *lactose,* the sugar in milk. Lactose is a combination of two sugar molecules, glucose and galactose. Before the intestines can absorb lactose, the double molecule must be split by the lactase enzyme present in the lining of the small intestines. Without this splitting action, the double molecule travels intact through the GI tract to the large intestine. There, bacteria cause the sugar to ferment, thus releasing hydrogen gas and drawing fluid osmotically through the intestinal walls into the bowel. The result is bloating, cramps, gas or flatulence, loose stools, or diarrhea. This problem is called either lactase deficiency or lactose intolerance, but it is not an allergy to milk and has nothing to do with fat content of milk—skim milk can cause as many problems as whole milk.

Except in rare instances, almost all babies are born with high levels of lactase in their intestines to digest milk. Lactase remains high throughout the first year or two of life, and then begins to drop off. In some people, usually as adults, lactase nearly disappears. It is very common for the body to lose its ability to manufacture lactase, and lactase deficiency eventually occurs in the majority of the world's population, particularly among American blacks, Native Americans, Jews, and Asians, groups that suffer a 70 to 80 percent incidence. Even though they experience uncomfortable symptoms, however, they are still able to derive some nutritional benefits from the fat and protein in milk products.

Not every adult becomes lactose intolerant. Northern Europeans and their American descendants and a few African populations seem to retain their ability to digest lactose even as they grow older. But it's also possible to have a lactase deficiency and not realize it. It sometimes sneaks up on people as they grow older. Symptoms of bloating and gas begin to occur gradually and you get used to it.

Roger Moore, a thirty-eight-year-old executive, was one of those people who had always had excessive flatulence, but for the last several years the condition had gotten progressively worse. When he came to see me he was at the point where he was afraid to go to a board meeting because of embarrassment about his noticeable symptoms. Roger avoided beans and other legumes like the plague, but his flatulence continued unabated. He occasionally had cramps in his lower abdomen and loose stools. His family doctor ordered x-rays of the upper and lower GI tract, which proved to be completely normal. Roger had recently traveled outside the United States, so a stool analysis for parasites was carried out, and that also proved to be negative.

Roger's father also had excessive gas, but it never seemed to bother him. The family just joked about it.

Roger was black, and this and his family history made me suspect he might be lactose-intolerant. He said he never drank milk, but after a little prodding he admitted he did use milk in his cereal and cream in his coffee. He was also an avid fan of ice cream. I was almost certain that he was lactose intolerant, but to prove it I performed a hydrogen breath test, in which a small tube is placed in the nostril and a quantity of exhaled air extracted. Air can be tested just as blood or urine can be analyzed. In this case, a gas chromatograph is used to analyze the air for excess hydrogen, which a lactose intolerant person will exhale after taking a dose of lactose.

Roger's test was distinctly abnormal. He was delighted to learn that simply avoiding milk products would cause a drastic reduction in his episodes of flatulence. He now uses lactase-added milk, and he can even eat ice cream if he swallows two tablets of lactase enzyme along with it. His father has started using lactase products too.

You can test yourself for lactose intolerance simply by drinking four glasses of milk on an empty stomach and waiting to see if any symptoms develop. Symptoms should appear within two to four hours. More sophisticated scientific tests are available to measure the increase in serum glucose after ingesting lactose by mouth (lactose tolerance test) or to measure the hydrogen content in your breath after ingesting lactose (breath hydrogen test), the test used for Roger.

For most people, lactose intolerance is not an all-or-nothing phenomenon. Many people can consume small amounts of milk or milk products and have no noticeable reaction. Most people with lactase deficiency have no trouble with the amount of milk that might be added to a cup of coffee, and they can often handle dairy products like yogurt, some cheeses, and butter. However, some people are so lactose intolerant that they must avoid all sources of lactose.

Lactose is in all forms of milk, including skim and low-fat milk products. For those people who need to consume low-lactose products there is lactase-added milk, acidophilus milk, and lactase drops and tablets (see Chapter 20).

11 Constipation

Constipation is a disorder in which there is difficulty in moving one's bowels. It is a common problem, particularly for those living in the Western hemisphere, and for some people it can be chronic and worrisome.

What is considered a "normal" bowel movement varies with the individual and geography. In the West, where diet tends to be low in roughage and fiber, stools tend to be low in weight; the normal number of bowel movements ranges from one movement twice a week to one or two movements a day. In Africa and other countries where grain is a dietary staple, movements are bulkier and much more frequent, as often as six or seven times a day.

Not everyone can or needs to have a bowel movement every day. Most people miss a day now and then and don't even notice it. However, for those who have chronic difficulty, who must strain to produce a dry, hard bowel movement, constipation can be uncomfortable and painful. Constipation often produces a bloated feeling because the bowel distends with gas and liquid, as well as large amounts of stool in the colon.

Causes

The most common cause of constipation is insufficient fiber in the diet, but many other causes can contribute to chronic constipation. People with IBS may have constipation because the colon doesn't always move naturally and spontaneously. Some medications may also cause constipation: iron supplements, antidepressant medications, painkillers, and some medications for hypertension. People suffering from low thyroid or an excess of calcium in the blood tend to suffer from constipation. So do pregnant women, and people who are sedentary or confined to bed rest. Depression at times can cause constipation. Travelers almost universally complain of constipation on the first few days of a trip, although it is difficult to say just why this is so. It may be change in sleeping or eating habits or water intake, or sitting long hours while traveling. Some people have a cathartic colon, or "lazy bowel," which means decreased bowel contractions often caused by excessive use of laxatives.

Some people develop constipation because they are too busy to move their bowels when they get the urge to defecate. Others may ignore the urge whenever they are outside their home. The longer the stool remains in the colon, the more water the colon reabsorbs. The stool gets smaller, firmer, and thus more difficult to evacuate. Over time, this disregard for the urge to have a bowel movement can interfere with the normal pattern of bowel habits and require relearning of the conditioned defecatory reflex.

Less commonly, constipation can occur when nerves to the bowel are severed during surgery. This can occur with some types of back surgery and after a hysterectomy. Bladder function may also be affected.

A word of caution about constipation: If you suffer from chronic constipation it's important to have a checkup to make sure no serious disease is present and that no underlying hormonal or electrolyte imbalance is causing the constipation. A *recent change* in bowel habits, especially a narrowing of stools, may signify serious disease and also requires a thorough evaluation. This is especially true when rectal bleeding is present. Any new onset of constipation, especially for those over age forty, should also be evaluated by a physician.

Treatment

Mildred Rosenberg was a seventy-two-year-old woman who had always had some degree of constipation. Recently, however, she noticed that her bowel movements were even less frequent, only once a week. It required a lot of effort to produce a few small, firm pieces of stool. The only way Mildred could have a larger bowel movement was to take Ex-Lax.

When we talked about her lifestyle, Mildred said that her arthritis had been getting worse, which had considerably slowed down her usual activities. At times she took aspirin with codeine for pain, but usually she took ibuprofen. She did not take any other medication. Her diet was noticeably deficient in fiber. There was no evidence of blood in her stool, weight loss, or any family history of colon cancer.

My impression was that Mildred had the same constipation she had had all her life, but that it was being made worse by inactivity and occasional codeine. To be certain no other problem existed, I ordered a barium enema and also examined her colon by flexible sigmoidoscopy. Both studies were normal.

The obvious treatment for Mildred was a change in diet. Because her diet was so low in fiber, I recommended one tablespoon of Metamucil and one glass of prune juice each day. She also began to add small servings of cereal, whole wheat bread, raw fruit, and vegetables to her daily diet, until after two weeks she was up to 25 grams of fiber a day. With this regimen she was able to have two to three well-formed bowel movements each week, without straining. This was a significant improvement for her (not everyone needs to have a bowel movement every day) and she did not require enemas, laxatives, or even stool softener.

Treatment of constipation depends on what's causing the problem to begin with. A change in drug therapy may be the answer for people who are on treatment regimens that produce constipation as a side effect. For most people, however, the answer will come from a change in diet, just as it did for Mildred.

Increasing fiber in the diet, in the form of fruits, vegetables, and grains, adds bulk and also increases the amount of water in the stool, which aids in its passage.

In most cases the Self-Help Nutritional Program, which recommends between 25 and 30 grams of fiber a day, is all that is necessary to treat constipation. Drinking plenty of water and getting regular exercise is also important. Runners often notice that they have a strong urge to defecate after a strenuous workout. For a quick fix, try that old standby prune juice. It works and it's good for you.

Bowel Retraining.   People who tend to ignore their body signals may over time have lost the ability to recognize when it's time to move their bowels. In this situation, it may help to go to the bathroom at the same time every day when a bowel movement is most likely to occur—usually about thirty minutes after breakfast or after a cup of caffeinated coffee (caffeine is a stimulant to the GI tract). Remember, however, that caffeine is a Flag Food for heartburn—again, what helps one GI problem may exacerbate another. (Nicotine, while a recognized colonic stimulant, is not recommended as a treatment for constipation or anything else.)

When you attempt to "retrain" your bowel, remember to take your time. Your mother may have told you to "do your business" quickly and get off the toilet, possibly to avoid hemorrhoids but probably because most of us grew up in a house with one bathroom. Today, even small houses usually have 2.5 bathrooms for the average 2.5-member families. So take your time.

If breakfast time finds you at work, any large meal will do for bowel retraining. When food enters your stomach it encourages the colon to contract. This impulse is transmitted by nerves that innervate the colon; certain hormones may also be involved. This reaction is called the gastrocolonic reflex. Some people, especially those with IBS, have an exaggerated gastrocolonic reflex—as soon as they eat they have to run to the bathroom. In bowel retraining the gastrocolonic reflex works in your favor.

Drugs. Scores of laxatives on the market can provide a quick fix to relieve constipation. They fall into several different categories according to their mechanism of action.

Bulk laxatives add volume and fluid to the stool. Metamucil, Effer-Syllium, and Perdiem are psyllium seed laxatives that add nonirritating bulk and promote normal elimination. FiberCon, which has a similar bulking action, contains the fiber calcium polycarbophil.

Stool softeners like Colace (docusate sodium) are not laxatives, but contain surface-active agents that help keep stools soft for easy, natural passage.

Magnesium salts like Phillips Milk of Magnesia and Haley's M-O work by increasing the fluid in the GI tract.

Stimulants like Ex-Lax and Correctol contain phenolphthalein, which stimulates intestinal water secretion and GI contractions. Dulcolax (bisacodyl) is a stimulant laxative that acts directly on the colon to make it contract.

In general, it is always best to try the gentlest agents first. Over time, harsh laxatives can damage the bowel and ultimately make you dependent on laxatives for bowel movement. For most people I recommend starting with a bulk agent or stool softener and, if necessary, adding a magnesium salt. Only in very difficult cases would a stimulant be the treatment of choice.

Enemas. Enemas, while not popular with most people, are safe and quite effective in treating constipation. A simple tap water enema can distend the rectum, simulating the normal stimulus that initiates defecation.

12 *Diarrhea*

In America we define diarrhea as stool output in excess of 300 grams (about three-quarters of a pound) a day, or an increase in the fluidity of stool. Diarrhea itself is not a disorder, but is a symptom of an underlying problem.

Causes

Diarrhea may be due to a disturbance in osmosis, secretion, or motility of the bowel; sometimes it is caused by a combination of two or more problems.

• Osmotic Diarrhea

The small and large intestines are lined with a semipermeable membrane. Fluid normally diffuses through the membrane and an equal pressure is maintained on either side. Food particles that cannot be absorbed by the intestines exert osmotic pressure and cause fluid from the bloodstream to cross the lining to try to balance the fluid concentration on either side. This excess of fluid in the intestine produces diarrhea.

People who frequently consume magnesium-containing antacids, such as Mylanta or Maalox, or laxatives, such as milk of magnesia, may suffer from osmotic diarrhea because magnesium cannot be absorbed by the intestine and will exert a strong osmotic force.

People who have a lactase deficiency (milk intolerance) also have problems with diarrhea. In this case, the milk sugar lactose cannot be absorbed. Bacteria in the colon break the lactose into simple sugars, which then exert an osmotic force on the colon, resulting in loose stools.

Fasting will generally improve osmotic diarrhea since the osmotically active agent will be eliminated.

• Secretory Diarrhea

As food passes through the GI tract, the cells lining the inside of the tube absorb fluid and nutrients and pass them into the bloodstream. These same cells also secrete fluid from the bloodstream into the interior of the tract.

Normally, the cells absorb much more fluid than they secrete, and there is a "net absorption." However, sometimes things can go awry and the cells secrete excessive fluid, causing a "net secretion"—and diarrhea. In this case, even fasting will not stop the diarrhea.

Certain bacteria such as cholera bacteria, Salmonella, and *Escherichia coli* (the cause of traveler's diarrhea) give off toxins that can stick to the intestinal lining. Although these toxins do not damage the intestinal lining, they do cause the cells to secrete massive amounts of fluid, which results in voluminous watery diarrhea typical of food poisoning. This is a common cause of acute severe diarrhea.

Some rare endocrine tumors give off hormones that act the same way as bacterial toxins. In this case, the diarrhea doesn't improve, and requires specialized treatments. A new drug Sandostatin is particularly effective in these difficult cases.

Any disease that damages the lining of the intestine, such as Crohn's disease, a common form of inflammatory bowel disease, tends to impair absorption and lead to net secretion and diarrhea.

• Motility Disorders

The normal contractions, or motility, of the small intestine act like a cleansing wave to prevent stagnation of fluid and overgrowth of bacteria. Certain diseases such as long-standing diabetes and scleroderma can affect the nerves and muscles of the intestine, so that bowel contents move sluggishly along the gastrointestinal tract, giving bacteria the opportunity to multiply. As bacteria compete for food they impair absorption of nutrients and can cause weight loss and diarrhea.

• Complex Causes

In certain instances, diarrhea may be caused by all of these problems working in unhappy concert. For the patient with Crohn's disease, for example, the last portion of the small intestine—the ileum—

is often inflamed *(ileitis)*. This means that bile from the liver cannot be absorbed normally and travels instead into the large intestine, where it stimulates secretion of fluid and leads to secretory diarrhea. Because the small intestine is inflamed, lactase production is impaired, which results in milk intolerance and loose stools (osmotic diarrhea). Prolonged inflammation can lead to scarring and the bowel can become obstructed, interfering with normal motility. (For such complex causes, treatment must also be diverse. In this particular case, drug therapy is needed to decrease inflammation, bind bile salts, and/or suppress bacterial growth.)

Most cases of diarrhea are not nearly so serious. Sudden onset of diarrhea associated with vomiting and cramping pains in the stomach is often caused by flu or other viruses.

Food poisoning, another common cause of diarrhea, is caused by bacteria, or toxins produced by bacteria, that have overgrown in food and find their way into the GI tract. Foods with high protein content —meat, chicken, fish, eggs—more readily support overgrowth of bacteria than carbohydrates do. Dry foods are also less likely to cause food poisoning. One important key to prevention is refrigeration. Food should never be allowed to sit out without refrigeration for more than three hours.

Just how severe these sudden attacks of diarrhea can be was illustrated by the famous airplane incident in the 1970s when a commercial airliner nearly ditched into the sea because everyone aboard, including the pilot, had eaten food overrun with Salmonella bacteria. The pilot had to overcome severe diarrhea and cramps to maneuver the plane onto the runway.

Treatment

With diarrhea of short duration there is no reason to initiate a diagnostic evaluation, unless you see blood in the stool or unless you have low blood pressure and become dehydrated.

Fluids. The most important action if you have an attack of diarrhea is to drink plenty of fluids to avoid dehydration. Gatorade is useful to replenish lost electrolytes such as sodium and potassium.

Diet. A clear liquid diet will sustain you until the bout of flu or food poisoning is over: bouillon, soup broth, carbonated beverages, fruit juices, and gelatin.

Avoid milk and dairy products since the milk sugar (lactose) may be poorly absorbed even in people who normally tolerate it well and thus worsen the diarrhea.

Drugs.   For the occasional bout, especially if you have IBS, over-the-counter remedies such as Pepto-Bismol, Kaopectate, and Imodium A-D may give symptomatic relief, but should not be used for more than two days without the advice of your physician. Diarrhea associated with IBS may be relieved by Donnagel, an antispasmodic and antidiarrheal agent.

Extreme Measures.   If a severe acute episode doesn't resolve itself within twenty-four to forty-eight hours, seek medical attention. People with fever or bloody diarrhea should consult their physician immediately.

Chronic diarrhea that lasts more than two weeks should be evaluated by your physician. Cultures will be taken and the stool analyzed for parasites. Your physician may also insert a tube called a sigmoidoscope into the rectum to examine the lining of the colon and take a bit of tissue for biopsy, and sometimes a barium enema or x-ray of the colon may be necessary.

Diarrhea Caused by Drugs

Many drugs such as antibiotics, heart medication (quinidine), ulcer drugs (Cytotec [misoprostol]), and others can cause diarrhea. If you are taking medication ask your doctor if it could be causing your diarrhea.

Antibiotics may cause diarrhea because they change the normal flora of the colon, permitting overgrowth of certain toxic bacteria. Mild diarrhea caused by antibiotics may be helped by Lactinex, a combination of *Lactobacillus acidophilus* and *Lactobacillus bulgaricus*. Usually the diarrhea improves by itself after stopping the antibiotic, but if it is severe or persists, consult your doctor. You may need a prescription for another antibiotic (vancomycin or metronidazole) to destroy the bacteria that are causing the problem.

Traveler's Diarrhea

The warmer and sunnier the climate of the country you are visiting, the more likely it is that you will develop traveler's diarrhea, the so-called Montezuma's Revenge so common in Mexico and Central

America. Travelers to the Middle East, Asia, and Africa are also vulnerable to traveler's diarrhea.

Symptoms are abrupt: watery diarrhea sometimes accompanied by disabling stomach pains and cramps. Fever, dehydration, nausea, vomiting, and prostration may all be part of the picture.

Whether you develop traveler's diarrhea does not necessarily depend on a roll of the dice. The illness is caused by ingesting toxigenic bacteria in contaminated water and food.

Food.   The best prevention is careful eating habits when traveling to endemic areas. Always drink bottled water, soft drinks, or fruit juices. Boiling water for five to ten minutes will kill the bacteria. But freezing water won't harm the bacteria, so forego ice cubes in your drinks.

The most common foods that get contaminated are vegetables and fruits. It may seem absurd to go to a tropical paradise like Mexico and pass up the beautiful fruits and vegetables. Washing fruit in local water obviously will not help. So, if you can't peel it, don't eat it. That means that lettuce is out, and avocados are in.

Hand to Hand.   Like the bugs that cause the common cold, harmful bacteria can be passed from hand to hand, or from money to hand. Wash your hands frequently when traveling and carry antiseptic towelettes to dry off.

Drugs.   If you follow these basic precautions you may be able to avoid traveler's diarrhea, or if you do pick it up your symptoms are likely to be mild. If it catches you, however, the best quick fix is Pepto-Bismol, and to a lesser extent Kaopectate, or Donnagel. Certain prescription antibiotics can also help. Make sure you follow the directions given on the labels and do not exceed recommended dosages.

Some travelers are not willing to risk coming down with traveler's diarrhea, which in its worst instances can be severely incapacitating. The attacks have ruined many expensive, long-planned vacations. One man I know had to be helicoptered off the beach in Acapulco and brought back to the United States for treatment. There are some prescription and OTC medicines you can take *before traveling* that will offer some protection against diarrhea. A word of caution: Even with preventive medication, you should still follow the precautions given above.

One of the most effective drugs is doxycycline, a long-acting antibiotic. Like many antibiotics, doxycycline can cause photosensitivity, which means that you are more likely to get sunburned. Since you are probably traveling in a sunny country, excess sun exposure can be a problem. Make sure you wear a high-rated sun screen (15 or above) and skip lying on the beach.

Trimethoprim sulfa (Bactrim DS), another effective antibiotic, produces a lesser degree of photosensitivity.

The idea behind taking antibiotics is to take them before you contract diarrhea. Waiting until you get traveler's diarrhea to start drugs gives unpredictable results.

Pepto-Bismol is the best OTC drug to prevent traveler's diarrhea. The bismuth in the product can suppress growth of bacteria, but it requires a lot of Pepto-Bismol to be effective as preventive treatment. A reasonable regimen is two tablets four times a day, starting twenty-four hours before you leave and continuing for two days after you return from your trip (as long as your overall use doesn't last longer than twenty-one days).

Pepto-Bismol contains salicylate, which like aspirin can cause ringing in your ears at high doses. If you experience this side effect, cut back on the dose until there is no more ringing.

13 Diverticulosis and Diverticulitis

Diverticulosis

Normally stool is pushed along as muscles in the colon wall contract in waves. Over the years little pouches may form along the outer surface of the colon wall. These outpouchings called diverticula (singular diverticulum) usually form at weak spots where blood vessels poke through the wall of the bowel.

Diverticulosis—which simply means having diverticula—is very common especially among older people, and often never causes noticeable problems. About 30 percent of Americans over age sixty have some degree of diverticulosis, and most of the time these diverticula cause no discomfort. But when problems do develop they can be painful and hard to treat. Sometimes the muscle in the colon walls thickens as a result of the high pressure necessary to push hard stool along. This can be associated with pain and spasm. Sometimes the pouches become infected, a condition called diverticulitis, or perforated, leading to severe abdominal infection and pain. Diverticula are the most common cause of bleeding from the lower GI tract.

Until recently, diverticulosis was treated with a low-fiber diet. Today, a high-fiber diet is considered a much more effective preventive treatment. Dietary fiber increases fecal bulk and softens stool; it also decreases the pressure inside the colon, and prevents formation of the pouches. Diverticulosis is seldom seen in vegetarians and is almost unknown in India and parts of Africa where a diet high in fiber is standard.

If you already have diverticulosis, the Self-Help Nutritional Program can help keep existing diverticula free of obstructions that can lead to infection (diverticulitis). Even mild increases in fiber intake can significantly improve stool bulk and softness.

Diverticulitis

Diverticulitis often occurs when an abscess or boil develops in the bowel wall. The infected diverticulum probably forms because dry hard stool or food matter gets stuck in the mouth or opening of the diverticulum. The usual symptoms of diverticulitis are fever and pain in the lower left side of the abdomen. Diarrhea and bleeding rarely occur with diverticulitis.

In an acute situation, a CAT scan may show a thickened colon wall or abscess cavity. An ordinary x-ray will help rule out perforation. The white blood count is often elevated in this condition. After the infection is treated and resolved, your physician will usually recommend a barium enema to confirm the diagnosis (but never during an acute episode).

Treatment of severe diverticulitis usually means hospitalization, with antibiotics and fluids given intravenously while the patient fasts in order to rest the bowel. Milder cases can usually be treated with a clear liquid diet at home and oral antibiotics. Chronic, recurrent attacks are usually treated surgically to avoid serious complications. Although fasting or clear liquids are useful and necessary during the acute phase of the illness, a high-fiber diet is the best long-term preventive course.

14   Hemorrhoids and Fissures

Hemorrhoids

Hemorrhoids are dilated, engorged veins in the rectum, which can protrude through the anus. Hemorrhoids are caused by increased pressure around the anus, often from chronic constipation, with straining to defecate, over months and years. Hemorrhoids are common in pregnancy. They also commonly accompany obesity. And some people simply have a natural predisposition to them.

Hemorrhoids may bleed, but often this appears as fresh, red blood on the toilet tissue, rather than as darker blood mixed with stool. See your doctor in either case. An examination of the rectum through a proctoscope or a colonoscopy is usually performed to exclude cancer. Mild cases of hemorrhoids can often be controlled by drinking fluids, eating a high-fiber diet, and having regular toilet habits. More severe cases can be very uncomfortable, and a wide variety of topical analgesics are used to soothe inflammation and relieve itching. Stool softeners and laxatives are also used for relief. Sometimes surgery is required to tie off the hemorrhoid.

Fissures

A fissure is a crack or tear in the skin of the anus, usually caused by constipation and straining to defecate. Sometimes they occur following anal surgery, proctitis, or other diseases. Since the surface of the skin at the anus has been broken, defecation irritates the fissure and may cause the sphincter muscle around the anus to go into spasm, resulting in intense pain.

Fissures can coexist with hemorrhoids, but there is no cause-and-effect relationship between the two conditions. Topical creams, stool softeners, and warm baths are used to ease symptoms. Some people resort to laxatives. And in severe cases, surgery may be required, but often is only partially helpful.

Treatment

The Self-Help Nutritional Program can go a long way to helping anorectal problems like hemorrhoids and fissures. The high-fiber program can prevent hemorrhoids and encourages hemorrhoid healing by improving stool bulk and intestinal transit time. It also softens stool and helps relieve constipation, prevent bleeding, relieve pain, and heal fissures.

Adding a bulking agent or stool softener to the diet twice a day is also helpful. Creams, foams, lotions, suppositories, or ointments can be soothing and promote healing when hemorrhoids or fissures cause pain and itching.

Here is a brief run-down on common OTC medications that can help hemorrhoids:

• Anusol-HC suppositories, like most hemorrhoid remedies, work by lubricating the swollen, irritated hemorrhoidal tissue. They also contain a mild analgesic. The dosage is given in the morning and at bedtime, and after each bowel movement. (Anusol-HC is a prescription-only drug because hydrocortisone is added to decrease swelling and itching.)

• Preparation H is available as suppository, ointment, or cream. This popular drug contains a live yeast cell derivative that supposedly helps build collagen and increases the ability of the tissue to absorb oxygen. Preparation H contains no anesthetic, but it does contain shark liver oil, which acts as a lubricant. Preparation H is applied whenever symptoms occur.

• Nupercainal (dibucaine) works primarily as a topical painkiller to relieve pain and itching. Nupercainal cream, ointment, or suppositories can be used whenever symptoms occur.

• Cortaid cream, ointment, or lotion contains 0.5% hydrocortisone to decrease inflammation of the tissues and relieve itching. It should not be used more than three or four times a day.

• ProctoFoam, a nonsteroid cream, contains pramoxine hydrochloride 1%, an anesthetic that sticks to the tissue lining and relieves pain and itching. ProctoFoam also lubricates the swollen, inflamed tissue and makes bowel movements easier. The dose is one applicatorful two or three times daily.

• Tucks pads, ointment, or cream contains witch hazel, which is soothing to inflamed tissues. It can be applied three to four times a day.

15 Inflammatory Bowel Disease
(Crohn's Disease and Ulcerative Colitis)

Crohn's disease and ulcerative colitis are potentially serious, progressive inflammatory conditions that usually involve the lower small intestine (Crohn's disease) and parts of the large intestine.

Crohn's disease is similar to ulcerative colitis, and it is sometimes difficult to distinguish between the two diseases. Symptoms of Crohn's disease and ulcerative colitis are similar—diarrhea, bloody stool, weight loss, and fever. Lower abdominal cramps—usually on the right with Crohn's, on the left with ulcerative colitis—are common.

Crohn's Disease

Crohn's disease can involve the gastrointestinal tract anywhere from the mouth to the perianal area. About 30 percent of people who suffer with Crohn's disease have inflammation only in the ileum—the last portion of the small intestine. About 55 percent have both ileal and colon involvement (ileocolitis), and 15 percent have only colon inflammation (Crohn's colitis). With Crohn's disease, inflammation extends through the entire wall of the bowel. The inflammation may cause the intestinal wall to thicken, and the inside diameter may narrow so much that an intestinal obstruction occurs.

About 30 percent of patients with Crohn's disease develop a fistula, an abnormal passage between two organs, or from an internal organ to the surface of the body. Internal fistulas may form between loops of intestine. External fistulas to the skin's surface—either the abdomen or the anal area—may be caused by the rupture of an abscess.

Abscesses form in about 20 percent of patients. Often, they occur around the anus, but some occur within the abdomen. Complications in other parts of the body may include inflammation of various parts of the eye, severe arthritis affecting various joints of the body, an inflammation of the spine, and skin disorders.

The cause of Crohn's disease is unknown. Some theories involve bacteria similar to tuberculosis bacteria, viruses, and immunological problems. Crohn's disease is not infectious, but it does appear to have a strong genetic tendency: in one study, about 40 percent of first-degree relatives of Crohn's patients developed inflammatory bowel disease. The genetic predisposition is not as great with ulcerative colitis.

Ulcerative Colitis

Ulcerative colitis is an inflammation of the colon and rectum that ultimately causes lesions or ulcers in the lining. Once established, the condition is always present, punctuated by sudden severe attacks. The inflammation involves only the lining of the colon, not the muscular wall underneath. Ulcerative colitis tends to involve the rectum (proctitis) and left colon, but may involve the entire colon (pancolitis). The cause of ulcerative colitis is unknown.

Fistulas do not form in ulcerative colitis, because the inflammation does not extend through the entire thickness of the bowel wall. Patients with colitis may also develop complications in other parts of the body, including arthritis of the spine and joints, skin ulcers and nodules, inflammation of the inner eyelids and whites of the eye, liver disease, and biliary tract disease.

Treatment

Diagnosis of these complex disease entities requires a full workup, including stool cultures, colon biopsy, and x-rays. Treatment for both diseases requires steroids or other drugs to decrease the inflammation. Drug therapy for Crohn's disease, especially ileitis, is usually stopped as soon as symptoms disappear; treatment for ulcerative colitis usually continues, in order to prolong remission of symptoms.

Even though many people can go for years without recurrent symptoms, medical management never completely cures these conditions.

Surgical intervention in ulcerative colitis, called colectomy, can be curative if the entire colon, including the rectum, is removed. This type of radical surgery, which usually leaves the patient with an ileostomy (the end of the ileum is sewn to the abdominal wall and a liquid stool empties into a plastic bag), is reserved for patients with severe disease that does not respond to medical management. Although few people with ulcerative colitis want an ileostomy, the adjustment is often easier than they expect and often they feel like a new person as they regain weight and strength.

Only 15 percent of Crohn's patients have purely colonic involvement; thus surgery to remove the colon usually does not cure the disease. The usual indications for surgery in Crohn's disease are obstruction, abscess in the area of the bowel, and formation of a fistula.

Obviously, the management and treatment of Crohn's disease and ulcerative colitis require careful medical supervision over the long term. The Self-Help Nutritional Program cannot necessarily be used as a treatment for either condition. Dietary management may be the *opposite*—a low-fiber, low-residue diet—especially when these diseases are in their acute phases. Patients are instructed to avoid fruits and vegetables, bran cereals and whole grain breads, seeds and nuts. A lactose-free and low-fat diet may also be important.

Once either disease is under control, the Self-Help Nutritional Program may help prevent symptoms of diarrhea, cramps, and perianal disease, which typically are part of these diseases. However, all dietary management for patients with inflammatory bowel disease should be carefully supervised by a physician.

Patients with ileitis may require iron and calcium supplements; if the inflammation is severe, trace metals (zinc, cadmium, chromium) must also be replaced. Patients with ileitis may need monthly shots of vitamin B12.

Ileitis sufferers tend to form kidney stones because of excessive absorption of oxalate. Dietary management includes a low-fat, low-oxalate diet (avoid spinach, rhubarb, and tea) plus calcium supplements (1 gram of calcium gluconate a day). This is one instance where extra calcium prevents kidney stone formation.

16 · Food Allergies

An allergy is an exaggerated reaction to a substance that in most people causes no response. The response is mainly to otherwise harmless substances: chemicals that come in contact with the skin; particles of dust or pollen that affect the respiratory passages or the surface of the eye; foods that affect the stomach and intestines.

Allergies are caused by a reaction of the immune system; they occur only on second or subsequent exposure to the offending agent, after the first contact has sensitized the body. Many common illnesses, such as asthma and hay fever, are caused by allergic reactions.

Many of my patients feel their GI symptoms may be caused by a food allergy. Symptoms of food allergies include nausea, vomiting, diarrhea, abdominal pain, indigestion, belching, rash, headache, runny nose, hives, asthma, and swelling of the face or throat. True food allergies are relatively rare in adults, however. Food allergies in infants and young children are much more common, possibly related to the introduction of solid food at too early an age, before the small intestine has had a chance to mature. Some allergies in children are caused by a protein in formula or cow's milk that is not present in breast milk. Many of us know of babies who require a soy-based milk because of milk allergy.

In adults, the symptoms that we loosely ascribe to food allergy may actually be related to disorders of the GI tract, such as IBS, peptic ulcer disease, gastroesophageal reflux disease, or inflammatory bowel disease.

Food Intolerance vs. Allergy

Sometimes what we think of as a food allergy is really a specific food intolerance. That may sound like splitting hairs, but a true allergy is a reaction to food mediated by your body's immune system. It tends to recur quite predictably each time you are exposed to the food, and symptoms usually begin soon after exposure, not several hours later.

A food intolerance, on the other hand, simply means that a particular food causes you some sort of distress. For instance, many people develop diarrhea, cramps, and flatulence after drinking milk. This is not an allergy, but rather an intolerance to milk because of a lack in the body of the enzyme needed to digest the milk sugar lactose. (When these symptoms occur in an infant, however, especially if a rash is also present, a true milk allergy is probably the cause because all infants have plenty of lactase to digest the milk sugar.)

Some patients say they are "allergic" to fatty foods because they have pain after eating foods that contain butter or cream. Most likely, they are suffering from gastroesophageal reflux or possibly from gallstones. Fatty foods tend to relax the LES valve between the stomach and esophagus, creating heartburn. Fatty foods also cause the gallbladder to contract, and if stones are present pain is the result.

Certain chemicals in food can also cause reactions similar to allergic responses. Histamine, a chemical released by specialized white cells in the body in response to an allergic reaction, can cause the flushing, itching, and hives characteristic of an allergic reaction. Certain foods, such as fermented cheese, pork sausage, canned tuna, and sardines, also contain histamine, and may produce in some people flushing, headaches, and a drop in blood pressure. Phenylethylamine, found in chocolate, aged cheese, and red wine, causes migraine headaches in some people.

Food additives can also cause problems. One common offender is monosodium glutamate, or MSG. A Chinese meal may have up to 2.5 grams of MSG, which can make susceptible individuals dizzy or short of breath. Some people have an asthmatic reaction to sulfites, which are often added to salads and vegetables to preserve a fresh appearance. Tartrazine in yellow food dye No. 5, often added to desserts, snacks, and drinks, can cause asthma, hives, and a runny nose. Nitrates found in smoked meat and cheese can cause GI upset, headache, and hives.

All of these are intolerances; none is a true food allergy. Those foods most likely to cause a true allergic reaction in adults are milk, eggs, nuts (especially peanuts), fish (especially shellfish), and wheat flour.

Diagnosis of Allergies

Unless the offending food causes a severe and immediate reaction, diagnosis of food allergy can be difficult. It may require a detailed list of foods consumed up to seventy-two hours prior to the reaction, as well as a detailed food record kept for at least two weeks correlating food eaten with symptoms.

If this fails to yield an answer, skin testing can be tried. This is the most reliable way of diagnosing food allergy, but it is by no means perfect. An extract of the food is injected under the skin; development of a red weal and flare means you are allergic to that food. Unfortunately, the test is not always accurate. Not only are there false-positive tests, but also false-negative tests (you have a food allergy, but the skin test is negative).

Sometimes the only way to accurately diagnose a suspected food allergy is to go on an elimination diet. You begin with a diet least likely to cause an allergic reaction—usually devoid of milk, eggs, nuts, and wheat products. If all goes well, you add specific foods to the diet, one at a time, with wide intervals between each addition, remaining alert for allergic reactions until the culprit is spotted.

Gluten-Sensitive Enteropathy

One food allergy that has been well studied involves gluten, a protein found in wheat. For those who are allergic to it, gluten can cause damage to the cell lining of the small intestine. The result is poor absorption of nutrients, greasy stools, weight loss, and diarrhea. Gluten-sensitive enteropathy is also known as sprue.

Removing gluten from the diet usually leads to prompt healing of the intestinal lining. Symptoms disappear, and the individual gains back the lost weight. Lactose may also need to be temporarily eliminated because the damaged cells temporarily lose their lactase enzyme activity.

Wheat is found in many products including bread, cakes, and pasta; gluten is also present in rye and barley and to a lesser extent oats. As you can imagine, a gluten-free diet is quite restrictive (see box). Fortunately, sprue is relatively rare, although in some areas of the world, especially Ireland and England, it is more common.

Food List for Gluten-Sensitive Enteropathy

The following is from the Thomas Jefferson University Diet Manual.

	Foods Allowed	*Foods Not Allowed*
Fruits	Plain fresh, frozen, or canned fruits	Fruits prepared with wheat, rye, barley, or oat products
Vegetables and Rice	Plain fresh, frozen, or canned vegetables and rice; homemade creamed vegetables if made with allowed thickeners	Vegetables prepared with wheat, rye, barley, or oats; commercially creamed vegetables
Soups	All soups prepared with allowed ingredients	Soups prepared with wheat, rye, barley or oats; canned soups (except clear broths); soup mixes; bouillon
Fats	Butter, margarine, lard, vegetable oils, shortenings (with no cereal starch added), cream, bacon fat, pure mayonnaise, homemade salad dressing, gravy and cream sauces prepared with allowed ingredients	Fats or salad dressings prepared with wheat, rye, barley, or oat products; salad dressing prepared from dry mixes; some brands of commercial mayonnaise
Desserts	Gelatin, homemade cakes, pies, cookies, if prepared with allowed flours; homemade cornstarch, rice, or tapioca puddings prepared with allowed ingredients	Commercial cakes, cookies, pies; certain brands of puddings, ice creams, sherbets, dessert mixes, custard mixes, and icing

	Foods Allowed	*Foods Not Allowed*
Sweets	Jellies; jam; honey; brown and white sugar; molasses; pure fruit syrup; some candy; chocolate; cocoa; coconut	Some commercial cakes
Beverages	Fresh brewed coffee, pure instant coffee or tea, Sanka, herb teas; Kool-Aid, carbonated drinks, fresh or frozen fruit juices, pure wine, brandy, rum, sake, tequila, vodka which does not have grain alcohol added (some "pop" type wines have grain alcohol added)	Postum; instant tea or coffee containing grains; fruit punch powders; beer; alcoholic beverages made from malt or grain, including blended whiskey and liqueurs, such as after-dinner drinks
Miscellaneous	Salt, pure ground peppers, herbs, cloves, ginger, nutmeg, cinnamon, chili powder, dry mustard, A-1 Steak Sauce, cornstarch, food coloring, bicarbonate of soda, cream of tartar, tomato puree, tomato paste, olives, pickles, cider vinegar, wine vinegar, rice vinegar, nuts, peanut butter made without additives	Some curry powders; chili seasoning mix; chutney; gravy extracts; meat sauces; certain brands of mustard, catsup and horseradish; soy sauce; Worcestershire sauce; chip and dip mixes; apple cider "flavored" vinegar; brewer's yeast; certain brands of peanut butter; products which contain monosodium glutamate (MSG), hydrolyzed vegetable protein, emulsifiers, starch, stabilizers, cereal fillers or thickeners, malt, or vegetable gum

17   *Stress: The Great GI Aggravator*

*T*ake my word for it, if you have a chronic digestive problem, stress is probably playing an active role in making your symptoms worse. Over the years there has been much controversy about whether stress actually causes GI problems. Many dozens of studies have been carried out trying to track down the origins of IBS, for example. Some findings support the idea that IBS is psychological in origin. Others find that IBS is a functional disorder aggravated by stress. If you have IBS, or any other digestive disorder, the important thing to know is that excessive stress increases your risk of an attack and is likely to make your symptoms worse. Tension, anxiety, worry, fear—all affect the GI tract. "I feel it in my gut" is one of the most common expressions in the American language, and we aren't joking when we say it. That's exactly where we feel it.

Our awareness of the effects of stress on the digestive tract began some 150 years ago when an American army surgeon was able to observe the stomach of a patient who had been wounded by a gunshot. The wound left a permanently opened passage between the stomach and the surface of the abdomen and gave the surgeon a clear view of the interior of the stomach. For many years afterward the physician made systematic experiments and observations of the digestive process in the stomach. He noted that when the patient was upset the mucosa, the coating that protects the stomach lining, changed color. The secretion of acids also increased and normal stomach contractions slowed down, so there was slower gastric emptying.

In the following decades many studies on both humans and animals were carried out, with similar findings. One famous observation was made by two physicians who were able to closely observe a man named Tom who lived most of his life with a gastrostomy, an artificial passage created between stomach and abdominal surface. For almost twenty years the physicians observed Tom and recorded their findings. When Tom was angry, they could see the stomach mucosa turn red, and acid secretions increased. If the disturbance was prolonged, severe pain was the result. When the patient was frightened, overwhelmed, or depressed, the mucosa turned pale, and the stomach contractions and secretions decreased.

These are only some of the ways our emotions affect our bodies. Our minds and our bodies interact at every level of our existence. Acknowledging the reality of the mind/body connection is essential to understanding overstress, which all of us experience at times, and to managing it, which few of us do very well.

As an example, a neighbor of ours who was plagued with irritable bowel syndrome had been an outpatient at Thomas Jefferson University Hospital for several months. She was enormously gratified with the results of changing her diet and took an interest in developing new recipes within the program's guidelines. Alice was one of our biggest success stories. Then one day she came in to see me with a full-blown attack of cramps and diarrhea. "I can't do the diet now," she told me. "I'm in the middle of getting ready for my daughter's wedding. We're expanding the office at work and I've got a big move scheduled. It's all just too much. Can you give me something just to get me through the next few weeks? I'm dying."

Alice was making herself sick. She was so busy at work that she felt anxious whenever she took time to meet with the photographer, the minister, and the caterer for the wedding. She needed to get her house cleaned before her relatives came to stay for the wedding weekend. Her daughter called her every five minutes with questions and new ideas. Alice was waking up several times a night with her mind racing and her heart pounding. At this point, she was having severe attacks of cramps and diarrhea several times a day. As a result, she was too harried to eat regular meals, let alone consider her diet.

Even if she had been sticking to the Self-Help Nutritional Program, however, it's likely that her IBS problems would have intensified. Alice's digestive upsets had always been aggravated by stress. She did not cause her own GI problem; the problem was probably the result of a number of factors, some of which may have been inherited. What Alice was not aware of, though, was how much she could help herself by understanding her body's individual response to stress. Learning to work with stress is a task for everyone, but it's especially important for people with GI problems.

Stress is produced by everyday events as well as by major life crises. It is experienced by everyone, but handled in different ways. Any event that requires us to adapt or change is a "stressor." We all feel best when dealing with just the right number of stressors in our lives. Too few and we become lethargic and bored; too many and we feel overwhelmed.

Stress that is managed well contributes to enhanced thinking and creativity, high energy level, endurance, and improved physical performance. Interest and productivity rise as stressors in our lives increase, up to a certain "just right" level. That perfect level is different for each of us.

Above that level, prolonged or frequent stressors begin to overtax our physical and mental resources, and our effectiveness decreases. Normal stress that continues without intervals for recovery develops into a state of overstress, and major body systems start to show signs of strain.

Overstress contributes to most of the major health problems in our culture, including heart disease, high blood pressure, arthritis, respiratory problems, cancer, and GI disorders. Stress tends to be most dangerous when it is cumulative, although for people with GI problems, even one significant stress event can trigger a reaction within twenty-four hours, if not immediately. When people are constantly faced with unrelenting stress over which they have little control, they simply may not have the biological resources to cope with it. If enough stressful changes are clustered together at one time, they leave people especially vulnerable to illness.

The Fight/Flight Response and GI Disorders

The "fight/flight response" is the body's reaction to any event that seems to demand some immediate action. It is a total psychophysiological response, involving body and mind, in which multiple body systems respond rapidly to the mind's perception of some demand or danger.

Our bodies are primed to take immediate action, to either fight off the threat or to flee it. Changes in the brain, nerves, heart, circulation, muscles, and GI tract are swift and effective. Following such an overwhelming response, recovery time may bring a sense of depletion or weakness ("Let me sit down and catch my breath"). If the body is not allowed adequate recovery time, the bodily systems suffer from overwork.

The GI tract responds at every level and in complex ways during the fight/flight response. Your mouth may become dry during a time of strain. Or your stomach may turn over from sudden anxiety. Or you may have the urge to defecate when facing a fearful event. Emotional states may change the acid balance in the stomach, or alter the normal contractions of the small and large intestines. Diarrhea results when contractions are too fast, and constipation when they are too slow. These stress-related changes can intensify existing GI imbalances, increasing discomfort and triggering attacks of cramps, diarrhea, constipation, or nausea. Perhaps worse is the slow, unseen damage done to the intestines by prolonged stress. When you are tense and unknowingly clench your jaws, your gut clenches, too. Some people sit for hours working under pressure with teeth tightly clenched, never realizing the pressure they're putting on internal organs.

The Three Sources of Stress

Stress overload is not usually the result of a single event, but of an accumulation of events. The degree of stress you feel stems from three different but interrelated sources.

• The Vagaries of Life

Pure external circumstances or life events cause stress. In any large group of people, more health problems are likely to occur for those who have recently experienced the greatest number of significant life events.

In their classic assessment of stress risks, Drs. Thomas H. Holmes and Richard H. Rake, psychiatrists at the University of Washington Medical School, interviewed nearly 400 people of various ages and backgrounds, asking each one to rank a series of life events on a scale of 1 to 100. At the top of everyone's list, with the highest impact of 100 points, was death of a spouse. Divorce ranked second in the line of stress. At the bottom of the list, but still considered stressful, were the Christmas holiday and traffic tickets.

In a later analysis of health statistics the researchers discovered that many widows and widowers died soon after losing the spouse. And divorced people immediately after their divorce were twelve times as likely to become ill as married or single people. A later study of 88 patients with major illnesses found that *93 percent* had suffered an accumulation of stressful life changes.

The critical finding of these investigators was that not only negative events were stress-provoking—all life changes, whether good or bad, created stress. From this work, stress came to be defined not as an event in itself, but as the product of change.

Life events have different stress "weight" for different people, but even welcomed, happy events, like a new and better job, are considered stressors. At any given time in your life, the more changes, challenges, losses, or additions you experience together, the more likely you are to develop stress-related problems. After such an accumulation, an interval of stability is needed for relief and to prevent illness.

Alice, for example, planned to sell her house and find another job right after her daughter's wedding. She would be wiser to put off these plans for a few months to give herself some recovery time from stress overload.

The daily little hassles of life can also be a potent source of stress: the car that won't start, the long line at the supermarket or the bank, the co-worker who interrupts constantly, the irate customer, the repair person who doesn't show up, the delivery van that never arrives.

Little hassles loom large on the stress front because you have so little control over them. They seem to attack in hassle squads, and some days you can handle them better than other days. This lack of control is significant, because frequent hassles define the most stressful jobs—jobs that combine a high degree of pressure with little control over decision-making. The person who works on the assembly line may have more stress than the CEO of a major corporation. Similarly, the average waiter (high pressure, low control) is under more stress than the average bank officer (high pressure, high control), the average forest ranger (low pressure, high control), or the average janitor (low pressure, low control).

In home life as well, the more control you have over your own life events, the less stress you feel. Furthermore, believing that you have control, even when you don't, can relieve stress.

• Your Personality

The second major source of stress is your own personality, including your natural temperament, your outlook on life, and your learned way of responding to events. Some people seem more "stress prone" than others, which may be partly a matter of innate biology. We know now that infants seem to come prepackaged with their own special temperament virtually intact. From birth, infants differ widely in how low-key or active they are, how bold or fearful, how irritable or placid. Life experiences interact with these innate differences to form more or less stable personality traits that persist throughout life.

Dr. Meyer Friedman, co-author with Dr. Ray Rosenman of *Type A Behavior and Your Heart*, first theorized that high-strung, anxious, "stressed out" people were more vulnerable to heart disease and elevated cholesterol levels than more relaxed individuals. In one well-known study, it was found that cholesterol levels of accountants rose significantly during the stressful weeks preceding April 15, and dropped back down to normal after the income tax due date passed. If your personality is bad for your health, however, you can often do something about it by changing your approach to life.

Overstress is often a product of our minds, of what we believe and how we imagine things to be. We live our lives by the rules of our perceptions and beliefs. Feeling overwhelmed, anxious, outraged, dejected, or hopeless is often a result of our reactions to our life circumstances, rather than the circumstance itself. And our reactions may be based on irrational beliefs that can trap us much more completely than external circumstances ever could. We actually have a great deal of power over our lives, because while we cannot always, or even often, control external circumstance, we do have a large measure of control over our own attitudes.

Alice, for instance, believed that it was entirely up to her to plan and carry off a perfect wedding for her daughter. She believed that it was a sign of weakness and incompetence to ask for help. She thought she was more comfortable if she had complete control of everything. No one told her this, but she believed it. It was up to her to please and satisfy everyone. She measured her success by the feedback she got from others. If she did not receive some sign of appreciation for her efforts every day, she felt dejected. The result of all this was that every detail of the wedding exposed Alice to the risk of feeling incompetent, guilty, a failure. Stress reverberated through her whole body, and her digestive system reacted to this emergency situation with alarm.

I have another patient who gets a similar kind of GI reaction, even though his personality is almost the direct opposite of Alice's. By his own admission, Harry is a fairly typical Type A personality—the person with "hurry sickness," a guy who first builds a pressure cooker and then lives in it. Harry runs his own mail order business, strives to achieve higher and higher levels of productivity every day, and tends to measure his worth in the number of sales he can make. Harry is outraged when other people fail to meet his own high standards; his blood pressure rises and his stomach churns with every delay in delivery, every clerical error, and any sign of slackening in his sales force. In fact, Harry is outraged all day long. He gets mad at trains that are late, cash machines that break down, and cars that don't jump forward the second the light turns green. Riding in the backseat of a taxi crawling through a traffic jam, Harry hyperventilated and had to get out and sit on the curb before he could get his breath back. He thought he was having a heart attack. Small wonder that Harry gulps antacids after meals, which he eats at his desk in between phone calls.

Given exactly the same stressful circumstance, Harry and Alice have different emotional responses. When Alice's train is late, she feels anxious and is afraid that she will fail to live up to someone else's expectations. When Harry's train is late, he feels angry and resentful, thinking he has been abused by someone else's incompetence. Alice holds some very harsh and rigid expectations for herself; Harry holds them for others. Both suffer unnecessary levels of stress without ever increasing their own effectiveness. And both experience that stress in their bodies.

These quick-trigger stress responses appear to be relics of childhood, when we first learned that it felt good if our parents approved of us, and bad if they didn't. Or when we thought other people were good if they fulfilled our wishes, and bad if they didn't. Often the response is based on false premises and negative thinking. We learn to react in preprogrammed ways. But just because these are old, old responses, which we have practiced faithfully for years, doesn't mean that we are stuck with them forever. Stress relief means recognizing not only the circumstances that cause us stress, but the *attitudes* that exacerbate them.

• Your Physical Self

The third component that determines how susceptible each of us is to stress overload is our individual physiology. Physiological differences influence how much privacy and quiet we need, how much stimulation, and how much predictability we need in our lives. For instance, some people are bored and depressed if they know exactly what's going to happen every day. Others must have routine to function at their best. Some people function best in a quiet environment, others thrive on having other people around. Each of us has a different pressure/performance curve. Some people can tolerate very high degrees of pressure before reaching peak performance. Others function best under mild or moderate pressure.

I think of one patient of mine, Nancy, who had just received a big promotion that should have pleased her very much. For years she had been in charge of planning and producing print materials for a large corporation. Even though she coordinated her work with that of other divisions in the company, she was largely autonomous in her job. A promotion to the customer service division, a job well within her abilities, brought her more prestige and money, but in the new position she had to supervise ten employees who handled customer complaints. Both employees and customers were often stressed out, presenting Nancy with one "people problem" after another. She began to have frequent attacks of heartburn and burning in the pit of her stomach. She woke up every morning dreading the day ahead. She longed to return to her solitary job in publications, and was convinced that she was weak because she couldn't tolerate the pressure of her new job. "You can't get anywhere in life if you can't take the pressure," she would say to me.

The fact is that stress is often the result of a mismatch between our temperament and the circumstances in which we find ourselves. For many reasons, some of which stem from her basic physiological temperament, Nancy is someone who does her best in a situation where she functions independently. I don't believe, as she does, that this is weakness of character on her part. In her previous job she had plenty of responsibility and plenty of other kinds of pressure that she handled well. The answer for Nancy may be to aim for a career move that allows her to function at her own personal peak performance.

A person's basic physiology also influences the way the body expresses stress overload. Some people have tension headaches, others have ulcer attacks. Some can't sleep at night, others have stomach cramps. Different people express stress in different ways. Nausea, heartburn, diarrhea, cramping, or constipation can all be responses to stressful situations.

An emotional response to overstress may also be rooted in physiology. You may have observed some people become very cool when stress seems overwhelming. Whether we become keyed up or detached, combative or timid, passive or hyperactive under stress may be tendencies built into our basic temperaments.

For example, people who often feel anxious or depressed may be victims of their biochemistry as well as their outlook on the world. When anxiety and depression appear to be important components of GI problems, psychotherapy may help. In a study of two groups of patients with irritable bowel syndrome, those who received psychotherapy improved both psychologically and physically, while the symptoms of those who received routine medical treatment either stayed the same or got worse. Because of the powerful link between body and mind, what we consider purely psychological realities can have real and measurable influences on the physical self.

Ways to Relieve Stress

Only in recent years have we been able to scientifically measure some of the effects of stress on our bodies and discover antidotes to its insidious work. Fortunately, the methodical study of stress overload has led to numerous successful ways to relieve damaging levels of stress. Here are some of the techniques that experts in stress reduction suggest:

• Reduce the amount of pressure in your external world. Try to identify the elements of a given situation that cause you to feel stressed. Then brainstorm a list of actions that you might take to either decrease the pressure or increase your sense of control. In every circumstance or life event there is always at least some small change you can make that will ease the stress for you.

Are You Stressed Out?

One of the problems with stress is that its effects are usually invisible—you can't see it, and you can't see what it's doing to your body until you become sick. And many of us don't know when we've had too much. I've noticed that people who are overstressed tend to lose touch with their bodies because one common reaction to stress is to become desensitized. Some physical signs of overstress are:

Digestive upsets of all kinds

Hair loss

Unexplained fatigue

Chronic body aches in the morning

Sleeplessness

Heart palpitations

Dizziness

Continuous sighing

Loss of appetite

Difficulty swallowing

Frequent urination

Rashes and itching

Some emotional signs of stress are:

Hair-trigger temper

Loss of concentration

Memory loss

Crying

• Is it lack of time or a too-tight deadline that is stressing you out? Can you manage your time differently in some way? Try saying no to new commitments until you feel less pressured.

• Are you overwhelmed by work and responsibilities? Try breaking down a big task into small steps, and take them one by one.

• Is an awkward or uncomfortable working or living space creating pressure for you? Can you change your physical environment?

• Is money a constant worry? Should you attend a seminar or course in personal financial management?

• When faced with a high-stress problem, remember to ask yourself, "Whose problem is this?" If the answer isn't yours, you may not have to solve it.

• In reading this chapter you have probably thought of hassles and stresses in your own life. Look back on some unwelcome event in your life, the memory of which still causes you anxiety and unhappiness—and find some way in which your life has been enriched because of it.

• Tackle harmful habits that undermine your health, especially smoking, drug use, alcohol abuse, and binge-starve patterns of eating. It's usually best to work on these one at a time, and to get professional help if you need it.

• Try to recognize when you are being negative and self-defeating.

• If stress and tension are chronic in your life, don't hesitate to seek professional counseling or therapy. It often takes someone else to help us identify the stress points and see a way out.

• All experts in stress relief advise that we should try for healthy balances in our lives. What they mean by this is balancing effort with rest, work with leisure, structured with unstructured time. Look for ways to restore the harmony between your body and mind.

• Take the time to pay attention to the quality of your life—with particular attention to nutrition and exercise. People who exercise regularly deal better with stress. They also sleep better and manage weight control better. Plan time for relaxation and pleasure, and stick to it. Some suggestions are a daily walk or an afternoon nap, daily relaxation exercises, regular workouts, and balanced, well-timed meals. All these activities can add harmony to life and keep moods on a more even keel.

Meditation and Relaxation Techniques

Relaxation can mean many things—yoga, meditation, deep breathing, or other relaxation methods. It can mean taking a long walk or counting backward from one hundred. Whatever form they come in, relaxation techniques can provide relief from stress by lowering blood pressure and heart rate. They also appear to reduce stimulation of gastric secretion and in general relax the gut.

In his landmark work, *The Relaxation Response*, Dr. Herbert Benson proved that meditation could help people who had high blood pressure because it produced a physiological response directly the opposite of "fight or flight." Meditating and other relaxation responses have been shown to decrease blood lactate, a substance strongly linked to anxiety. During the first ten minutes of meditation, blood lactate levels drop rapidly and remain extremely low throughout meditation. This effect may block the stress mechanism that some researchers believe to cause many different ailments.

Relaxation techniques have also been shown to help regulate glucose in some people with adult-onset diabetes, to open constricted air passages in those with chronic, nonseasonal asthma of the upper airways, and to lower elevated cholesterol levels.

Regular exercise workouts also provide great release from stress. The endorphins released into the bloodstream during strenuous exercise create an almost palpable sense of well-being.

The trick to stress relief is to find a relaxation technique that's right for you and fits into your lifestyle.

Part Three

Quick Fixes with OTC Products

*E*veryone and anyone can have a sudden GI problem —from simple indigestion to diarrhea and vomiting. People who have chronic GI problems may have a sudden flare-up of their symptoms even when they follow the Self-Help Nutritional Program. So it's good to know how to help yourself get immediate relief from a sudden attack.

Unfortunately, many of the traditional remedies believed to aid digestive upsets may actually make things worse for GI patients. For example, swallowing a bubbling, aspirin-containing Alka-Selzer for an upset stomach can irritate the stomach lining and make ulcer patients suffer.

Using OTC Products

Over-the-counter (OTC) drugs, like prescription drugs, have benefits as well as potential problems. OTC drugs are easy to purchase and, when used appropriately, can often provide some relief of GI problems. Drugs often become OTC by lowering the dose of a prescription drug, however, which usually makes them safer, but also makes them weaker and less effective. There are many OTC drugs on the market that either have no efficacy in treating a particular disease or are labeled "possibly effective."

Unless an OTC drug has been recommended by your physician, it's up to you to diagnose your problem correctly and then choose the best OTC drug to treat it. There is a lot of room for error in this method, and OTC drugs can cause problems. Even though weaker than prescription drugs, OTC remedies can still have side effects, and may even lead to life-threatening complications in people with GI problems. For instance, aspirin and nonsteroidal anti-inflammatory drugs (NSAIDs) like ibuprofen can cause serious ulceration of the stomach lining and lead to gastrointestinal bleeding.

All in all, self-diagnosis and drugs of any kind make a bad combination. If you have GI symptoms you should always be evaluated by a physician. Based on the diagnosis, your physician can advise you about which OTC drugs will be most helpful for you if you need them.

That said, many people are still going to purchase OTC medications to relieve symptoms. Here is some information about common OTC medicines and their effect on GI disorders.

Over-the-Counter Remedies

• Antacids

Antacids, commonly used to help relieve heartburn, are one of the most widely used OTC drugs on the market. Antacids work by neutralizing stomach acids and can also relieve gas pains when they contain simethicone. Antacids are also used to treat peptic ulcer disease. Recent data shows that even low doses of antacids heal duodenal ulcers as well as the prescription drugs usually prescribed for ulcer treatment (Tagamet, Zantac, Pepcid, Axid, or Carafate).

Antacids come in tablet or liquid form. We used to recommend liquid over tablets because liquids had a better neutralizing capacity, but newer tablet formulations are nearly equivalent in their capacity to neutralize acids, so the two preparations can be used almost interchangeably.

All antacids work the same way, but different products contain different ingredients. Both tablets and liquids contain either magnesium, aluminum, calcium, or a combination. There can be some side effects when these products are used on a regular basis.

Magnesium-containing antacids (for example, Maalox or Mylanta) taken frequently may cause diarrhea. Those containing aluminum, such as ALternaGEL, may cause constipation. I usually recommend that my patients who take antacids regularly alternate one with another to offset the potential side effects of each.

Theoretically, calcium-containing antacids have the potential to stimulate more acid secretion over the long run. But women who would like extra calcium to help prevent osteoporosis might prefer calcium-containing antacids like Tums or Titralac. The best advice is to experiment with various products and discover which ones seem to work best for you without producing side effects.

Antacids come in regular strength and extra strength. Extra-strength preparations (often represented by the Roman numeral II after the name) should be used only when the recommended dosage of regular antacid does not fully control symptoms. The equivalent volume of an extra-strength preparation will produce a greater incidence of side effects such as diarrhea and constipation.

Some brands of antacids that carry the suffix *Plus*—for example, Maalox Plus—contain simethicone, which absorbs gas. People who suffer from gas pain are often helped by simethicone-containing antacids. Simethicone is also available without an antacid (Mylicon) for people who suffer from gas but not acid-related problems.

People who suffer from intermittent heartburn take antacids on an "as needed" basis. This is a good idea if your heartburn is usually well managed on the Self-Help Nutritional Program but you still experience occasional heartburn. In general, full doses of antacids should not be taken for more than two weeks without your physician's advice. People who have any kind of kidney disease should not take antacids except under a doctor's supervision.

If you take antacids as the primary treatment for ulcers, then you must take them on a regular basis, even if you don't have pain. The best time to take antacids this way is one hour after meals and at bedtime, but not at the same time as other medications because the antacids may alter the body's ability to absorb certain drugs.

If you use antacids to supplement other forms of ulcer therapy, take them only when you need pain relief.

• Pepto-Bismol

One of the most versatile of all OTC products, Pepto-Bismol can soothe heartburn and indigestion as well as help settle an upset stomach and ease nausea. It is widely used to control routine diarrhea, as well as traveler's diarrhea, and has recently been used to treat duodenal ulcers that do not respond to usual anti-ulcer medication. (The active ingredient in Pepto-Bismol is bismuth subsalicylate, which appears to suppress the growth of bacteria, particularly *Helicobacter pylori*, often found in the stomach in patients with duodenal ulcers.)

• Pain Relievers

Even though many GI diseases cause pain, pain relief is often achieved without traditional painkillers. For example, antacids relieve the pain of heartburn and ulcers better than painkillers. An antispasmodic such as Bentyl or Pro-Banthine, both prescription drugs, probably works better than aspirin or acetaminophen for the pain associated with attacks of IBS.

However, people with GI conditions occasionally suffer from other kinds of pain—headaches, joint pains, muscle aches—that are best

Quick Fixes with OTC Products

When using any OTC or prescription medication, read the instructions and package insert carefully before using. The dosage recommendations given here are typical for the average person. Pregnant women should not use any medication without the advice of their physician.

Symptom	OTC Remedy	Dosage
Gas pain (without heartburn)	Mylicon	1–2 tablets, 4 times a day, after meals and at bedtime
Gas pain (with heartburn)	Maalox Plus Mylanta Plus	1–2 tablets, 4 times a day, after meals and at bedtime
Heartburn	Antacid tablets or liquid	2–4 teaspoons liquid or 2–4 tablets, between meals and at bedtime
Heartburn not relieved with regular antacids	Extra-strength Maalox or extra-strength Mylanta	1 hour after meals, at bedtime, and as needed
Traveler's diarrhea, treatment	Pepto-Bismol	2 tablets or 2 tablespoons liquid, 6 times a day
Traveler's diarrhea, prevention	Pepto-Bismol	2 tablets, 4 times a day, beginning 24 hours before trip, continuing 2 days after return, not to exceed 21 days total
Ulcers (unresponsive to anti-ulcer medication)	Pepto-Bismol (plus antibiotic)	2 tablets, 4 times a day, for 3 weeks

Symptom	OTC Remedy	Dosage
Constipation	Metamucil or Effer-Syllium or Perdiem	1 tablespoon, twice a day
Headache	Tylenol	2 tablets, every 4 hours as needed
	Extra-strength Tylenol	2 tablets, every 6 hours as needed
IBS		
Diarrhea	Pepto-Bismol	Same as for traveler's diarrhea
	Imodium A-D	4 teaspoons after first loose BM, followed by 2 teaspoons after each subsequent BM (do not exceed 8 teaspoons/day)
	Kaopectate	4–8 tablespoons after each loose BM
Constipation	See above (Constipation)	
Cramps	No effective OTC products. Ask your physician about Bentyl or Donnatal.	
Hemorrhoids	Anusol H-C	1 suppository, a.m. and p.m., after each bowel movement
	Preparation H or Nupercainal	As needed
	Cortaid ProctoFoam Tucks	3 or 4 times a day

helped by painkillers. What kind of painkiller can you use that won't make your GI problem worse?

Two common painkillers are aspirin and nonsteroidal anti-inflammatory drugs (NSAIDs) such as ibuprofen, found in Advil, Nuprin, and several prescription drugs. (When NSAIDs are taken in low OTC doses of 200 milligrams they lose their anti-inflammatory action but are still effective pain relievers.) Both OTC and prescription doses can damage the stomach and to a lesser extent the duodenum.

The cells that line the stomach are normally in a very hostile environment, but have a mucosal defense against the acid and pepsin that constantly bathe the stomach lining. A group of fatty acid derivatives called prostaglandins, naturally present in the stomach lining, help make the extra mucus and bicarbonate necessary for this protective defense system. Both aspirin and NSAIDs block the production of prostaglandins so that the mucosal defense weakens, and ulcers may form. As a result, people who already have upper GI problems, specifically ulcers, are at even higher risk of suffering complications. Other people at risk are those over sixty years of age, women, those taking steroids plus NSAIDs, smokers, and those with rheumatoid arthritis. Even buffered or enteric-coated products do not fully protect the stomach. So if you have upper GI problems, you should avoid aspirin or NSAIDs if possible.

One alternative is acetaminophen (Tylenol), which is a painkiller that does not irritate the stomach lining. Even acetaminophen has drawbacks if overused, however. In massive doses it can cause serious liver damage. High but conventional doses taken over a long period of time can also damage the liver, especially if you also consume excessive amounts of alcohol. The damaging effects of Tylenol and alcohol appear to be cumulative, so if you take Tylenol on a regular basis it's important not to drink. As long as you avoid alcohol and take no more than 4 grams of Tylenol a day, it's unlikely that you will suffer any kind of liver damage (two extra-strength Tylenol equal 1 gram).

One problem is that Tylenol is not anti-inflammatory, and while people do take it for arthritis, it is not as effective as aspirin or NSAIDs in high prescription doses. If you have an upper GI problem and you need aspirin or NSAIDs for arthritis, ask your physician about a relatively new drug called misoprostol (Cytotec). Misoprostol is a synthetic prostaglandin that reverses the hormone deficiency caused by aspirin and NSAIDs and prevents injury to the stomach. Misoprostol is taken concurrently with aspirin or NSAIDs. Women over age sixty who take aspirin or NSAIDs for rheumatoid arthritis are at risk for developing ulcers, especially if they also smoke. They may benefit particularly from misoprostol. Other standard ulcer drugs (Zantac, Tagamet, Carafate) offer the stomach little or no protection from aspirin and NSAIDs but do protect the duodenum.

Part Four

The Self-Help Nutritional Program:
The Two-Week Master Program

*T*he Self-Help Nutritional Program for GI disorders uses state-of-the-art information to create a nutritional plan that can be used by almost everyone with GI problems.* It brings together in one program all the knowledge gained in the past two decades about how food behaves and reacts within the gastrointestinal tract.

The Two-Week Master Program

In a standard American diet, 35 to 45 percent of the daily calories come from fat; 12 to 20 percent from protein; and 40 to 50 percent from carbohydrate. In the Two-Week Master Program the goal is to shift the emphasis of your diet so that less than 30 percent of daily calories come from fat; 12 to 20 percent come from protein; and 55 to 60 percent or more come from carbohydrates.

The Two-Week Master Program will help you choose foods that offer good nutritional value for the calories, while steering clear of the foods that create problems for you.

Food has seven constituents: proteins, fats, carbohydrates, fiber, water, vitamins, and minerals. The program contains all seven constituents in the amounts necessary for good health. At the same time it provides them in a balance that the digestive tract can handle without stress.

In my years of working with patients suffering from GI problems of all kinds, and also with overweight patients, I've learned a great deal about what *doesn't* work as far as diets are concerned. My patients have told me time and again that they are discouraged by complicated diets. They don't want to look up calories or memorize food exchanges. And they don't want to face the same boring food day after day.

---

* The program is not recommended for people with acute diverticulitis or moderate to severe inflammatory bowel disease (Crohn's disease, ulcerative colitis) unless directed by a physician.

With that in mind, and with the help of Cheryl Clifford Marco, R.D., I've tried to make the Master Program as simple as possible and as delicious as possible. By offering varied menus, the program avoids the spartan and monotonous fare that has characterized nutritional treatment of GI disorders in the past. These menus will quickly disprove the idea that foods easy on your digestive system must necessarily be bland and boring. If you cannot imagine life without Mexican food or other colorful, entertaining menus, all is not lost. The best part of this program is that it's made up of foods that everyone else eats. In the surprised words of one of my patients, "I'm finally eating real food again!"

The Two-Week Master Program uses many of the recipes in this book, as well as everyday foods that you are probably accustomed to eating. It may seem that you will have to learn a lot of new recipes, but most of them are simple and quick, easy to learn and easy to remember. A little organized shopping will put you in a position to prepare all of them.

• About the Recipes

The recipes in the last section of this book have been designed for quick and easy meal preparation. With a little practice you will be able to prepare them automatically without even looking at the book. To ensure good results, every recipe has been carefully kitchen-tested and retested several times during development.

On many days, you will eat animal protein only once, and the portions are smaller than what you are probably accustomed to. Be assured that your diet is nutritionally balanced and that you are getting more than enough protein on any given day.

To help you calculate, every recipe contains the following nutritional information.

Calories Per Serving.   Most recipes are for four servings, but all indicate their yield.

Percent of Carbohydrate.   This is the percentage of calories derived from carbohydrate. Overall, the meal plans are designed to be high in carbohydrate: 55 to 60 percent of your total daily calorie intake should be derived from carbohydrate. Some recipes are almost all carbohydrate, although others are fairly low.

Percent of Protein.   This is the percentage of calories derived from protein. About 12 to 15 percent of your total daily calories should be derived from protein. Although this is probably less animal protein than you are accustomed to eating, it is more than enough for the average man or woman.

Percent of Fat. This is the percentage of calories derived from fat. Less than 30 percent of calories in the diet are derived from fat. Although the fat content of the diet is low overall, some individual recipes are higher than others. A good rule of thumb when purchasing prepared foods is to buy products with no more than 3 grams of fat per 100 calories.

Grams of Fat. This is the total grams of fat per serving. There are 9 calories in 1 gram of fat. Some recipes appear to have a high percentage of fat calories, but because total calories are so low, the grams of fat are also quite low. This is particularly true of the salad recipes, which are predominantly low-cal vegetables, but have some oil or mayonnaise in their dressings.

Grams of Fiber. This is the total grams of dietary fiber per serving. It is recommended that 20 to 30 grams of fiber be consumed daily.

• How Many Meals a Day?

Three standard meals a day is the way to go for most people with GI disorders. However, certain conditions may benefit from several smaller meals each day.

People who have had stomach surgery for peptic ulcer disease may find that since they no longer have a pyloric sphincter, which controls the amount of food from the stomach that enters the small intestine, a large volume of food is deposited into the small intestines at once. This "dumping syndrome" can cause several problems, including diarrhea, too rapid absorption of glucose, excessive insulin release, and low blood sugar a few hours after the meal. Some people with long-standing diabetes fill up easily and are unable to eat large meals. And some people with IBS, especially those who have an exaggerated, almost uncontrollable urge to move their bowels after a meal, do much better if they eat smaller meals. For these people, breaking the three basic meals into smaller units and eating several times a day may be helpful.

A word of caution: At no time should you eat *fewer* than three meals a day.

• Snacks between Meals

Snacks are not included in the meal plans, and for most people they will be unnecessary. If you are interested in adding snacks to the basic meal plan, make sure you stay within the recommended guidelines of the diet. Also, if you have difficulty eating the recommended portions at one sitting, you can stretch the same amount of food into five or six smaller meals. Remember, though, that snacks should not be eaten in the evening or just before bedtime because food late at night can increase GI distress.

• Beverages

Noncaloric soft drinks are not included in the meal plans, but you may have them if you wish. If your GI complaint permits it, coffee and tea may be used (see Chapter 24). Water is probably the best beverage you can drink with your meals, or at any other time.

Whenever milk is specified in a meal plan, it is 1% low-fat milk. You may substitute lactose-free low-fat milk products in any of these menu plans (see Chapter 31).

After Two Weeks

The Two-Week Master Program gives you macronutrient values (for protein, carbohydrate) as well as fiber and calorie values for each recipe and meal plan. This means that after you have followed the program for two weeks you can begin to pick and choose recipes that personally appeal to you, and also suit your particular requirements. You can also begin to invent or adapt your own recipes, using the guidelines set out in the chapters that follow.

Overall, the Self-Help Nutritional Program for GI disorders is so normal that you will be able to incorporate its nutritional guidelines easily into your family's lifestyle.

Once you have completed the Two-Week Master Program, the recipes are intended to become a part of your everyday cooking for yourself, for family, and for friends. It's important that everyone in your family can enjoy the same food. The tenets of the program are good for all ages—reduced fat and cholesterol, increased complex carbohydrates. Just as important to you and your family, these recipes taste good, provide variety, and are nutritionally sound. Eating habits are formed early in life. When you choose a healthy diet for yourself to help your GI problems, you can be assured you are also having a positive impact on the health and lifestyle of others you live with, including children.

It may seem hard to shift from old eating habits to a new style of eating. Change is never easy. But in this case changing your diet will bring you immediate rewards. You will begin to feel better and find relief from discomfort that may have been going on for years.

Even George, the attorney who needed his mother to help him through the Two-Week Master Program and who didn't know a pot from a potato, was able to stay with the diet because it helped him make a gradual shift in his eating habits. After following the Two-Week Master Program fairly rigidly, he returned to his old eating habits—with some important changes. He cut down on spices, fats, and regular milk products. Then he tried preparing a couple of the recipes himself. He paid more attention to what he was doing and increased his repertoire. Within a few weeks, the benefits of the new program had begun to settle in and he found he had made the transition.

The key to good nutrition is flexibility. Any nutritional plan should become an integral part of your overall lifestyle. Whether you grab lunch in a diner or dine in a four-star restaurant, you should still be able to stick to the fundamental principles of this program. The idea is to choose foods that offer good nutritional value for the calories, while steering clear of the foods that create problems for you. If you follow the six principles of the Self-Help Nutritional Program, you should succeed in mastering your GI complaint.

High fiber, low fat, low lactose, low spice, low gas-forming foods, and low calories: it's important to understand the principles behind each of these concepts before incorporating them into recipes and menu plans. These are the six elements that you will use every day for the rest of your life.

The program that follows contains an average of 1850 calories a day. Some people will need more calories and some less, depending on their height and body build. See Chapter 26 for information about adjusting the calorie content of the program to your needs.

Menus

Day 1   1735 calories
54 grams of fat (28% of calories)
29 grams of fiber

BREAKFAST   *Frosted Melon Cooler
                2 slices whole wheat toast
                2 teaspoons margarine or butter
                1 tablespoon jelly or jam

LUNCH   2 whole wheat pita pockets stuffed with
                1 cup or more fresh vegetables, such as grated
                   carrots, bean sprouts, cucumber, pepper and
                   tomato
                2 ounces grated cheese
                *2 tablespoons Basic Vinaigrette Dressing
                1 cup 1% low-fat milk

DINNER   *Sweet and Sour Shrimp
                1 cup noodles, preferably whole wheat
                *Snow Pea Salad
                1 kiwi, ½ cup raspberries

Day 2   1934 calories
47 grams of fat (22% of calories)
22 grams of fiber

BREAKFAST   *Orangy French Toast
                1 cup 1% low-fat milk

LUNCH   *Eggless Salad
                2 slices whole grain bread
                1 pear

DINNER   *Marinated and Grilled Chicken Breast
                *Potato Salad
                Tossed green salad
                *2 tablespoons Basic Vinaigrette Dressing
                *Blueberry Apple Crumble

Day 3   1846 calories
50 grams of fat (25% of calories)
29 grams of fiber

BREAKFAST   *Blueberry Apple Crumble (leftover from Day 2)
                ½ cup plain low-fat yogurt
                1 cup 1% low-fat milk

* Asterisk indicates a recipe you will find in Part Eight.

LUNCH   *Rice Salad
2 whole wheat rolls
2 teaspoons margarine or butter
1 popsicle
1 orange

DINNER   *Marinated and Grilled Flank Steak
*Eggplant in Rich Tomato Sauce
*Cold Barley Salad
1 whole wheat roll
1 teaspoon margarine or butter
*Banana Dream Pie

Day 4

1814 calories
42 grams of fat (21% of calories)
31 grams of fiber

BREAKFAST   2 cups whole grain cold cereal
1 cup 1% low-fat milk
½ cup blueberries
1 slice whole wheat toast
1 teaspoon butter or margarine

LUNCH   *Marinated and Grilled Flank Steak (leftover from
Day 3) on
2 slices French bread
1 tablespoon catsup
½ cup applesauce

DINNER   *Acorn Squash Soup
*Chicken and Herbs Baked in Foil
*Kasha and Corn
Tossed green salad
*2 tablespoons Basic Vinaigrette Dressing
1 banana

Day 5

1748 calories
50 grams of fat (26% of calories)
26 grams of fiber

BREAKFAST ½ melon
1 cup oatmeal
1 cup 1% low-fat milk
2 slices whole wheat toast
2 teaspoons of margarine or butter
1 tablespoon jelly or jam

LUNCH *Acorn Squash Soup (leftover from Day 4)
1 bagel
1 tablespoon cream cheese
½ cup pineapple (packed in its own juice)

DINNER *Veal with Sun-Dried Tomatoes
*Lemony Potatoes
Tossed green salad
*2 tablespoons Basic Vinaigrette Dressing
*Patriotic Pizzazz

Day 6

1834 calories
42 grams of fat (21% of calories)
22 grams of fiber

BREAKFAST *Strawberry Pancakes
2 teaspoons margarine or butter
3 tablespoons maple syrup
1 cup 1% low-fat milk

LUNCH *Beautiful Bow Tie Pasta
1 whole grapefruit

DINNER *Flounder in a Flash
*Cinnamon Rice
*Broiled Tomato Halves
Tossed green salad
*2 tablespoons Basic Vinaigrette Dressing
*Apricot Apples

Day 7

1778 calories
53 grams of fat (27% of calories)
24 grams of fiber

BREAKFAST *Granola Cereal
½ cup strawberries
1 cup 1% low-fat milk
1 slice whole wheat toast
1 teaspoon margarine or butter

LUNCH   *Tuna Patties on hamburger roll
            1 peach
            2 plums

DINNER   *Oriental Barbecued Chicken
            *Veggie Stir-fry
            *2 slices Easy Cornbread
            *1 Peanut Butter Bar

Day 8   2011 calories
            52 grams of fat (23% of calories)
            24 grams of fiber

BREAKFAST   ½ melon
            *2 Oatmeal Raisin Muffins
            2 teaspoons margarine or butter
            1 cup 1% low-fat milk

LUNCH   *Turkey Meatball Soup
            *1 slice Easy Cornbread (leftover from Day 7)
            *1 Peanut Butter Bar (leftover from Day 7)
            1 cup 1% low-fat milk

DINNER   *Fettuccini with Clam Sauce
            1 whole grain roll
            1 teaspoon margarine or butter
            *Spinach Salad
            1 peach

Day 9   1978 calories
            46 grams of fat (21% of calories)
            29 grams of fiber

BREAKFAST   *Hot Buckwheat Cereal
            1 slice of whole wheat toast
            1 teaspoon margarine or butter
            1 tablespoon jelly or jam
            1 cup 1% low-fat milk

LUNCH   *Fettuccini with Clam Sauce (leftover from Day 8)
            1 whole grain roll
            1 teaspoon margarine or butter
            1 banana

DINNER   2 baked pork chops
              *Boiled Potatoes with Apples
              *Cucumber-Radish Salad
              *2 Oat Biscuits
              1 orange

Day 10   1857 calories
             46 grams of fat (22% of calories)
             26 grams of fiber

BREAKFAST   *Fruit Cup
              1 bagel
              1 tablespoon cream cheese
              1 tablespoon jelly or jam

LUNCH   *Fruited Chicken Salad
              2 whole wheat pita pockets
              1 cup 1% low-fat milk

DINNER   *Teriyaki Salmon Kabobs
              1 cup brown rice
              *Apple Salad
              *4 Oatmeal Drop Cookies

Day 11   1847 calories
             59 grams of fat (29% of calories)
             24 grams of fiber

BREAKFAST   *Tomato, Mushroom, and Basil Omelet
              2 slices whole wheat toast
              2 teaspoons margarine or butter
              1 tablespoon jelly or jam
              1 cup orange juice

LUNCH   2 cups whole wheat spaghetti with
              1 cup chopped fresh vegetables, such as carrots,
                 peppers, tomatoes, zucchini, mushrooms
              *2 tablespoons Basic Vinaigrette Dressing (over
                 pasta and vegetables)
              *2 Oatmeal Drop Cookies (leftover from Day 10)

DINNER   *Lemonade Chicken
              *Vegetable Kabob
              *Cold Bulgur Wheat Salad
              *Fruit Cup (leftover from Day 10)

Day 12 1915 calories
50 grams of fat (23% of calories)
30 grams of fiber

BREAKFAST ½ grapefruit
*3 slices Banana Bran Bread
1 cup 1% low-fat milk

LUNCH *Wheat Berry Salad
1 whole wheat pita pocket
1 banana

DINNER *Salmon Mousse on 4 slices cocktail rye bread
*Creole Topped Potato
Tossed green salad
*2 tablespoons Basic Vinaigrette Dressing
1 whole grain roll
1 teaspoon margarine or butter
½ cup sherbet

Day 13 1820 calories
49 grams of fat (24% of calories)
25 grams of fiber

BREAKFAST *Lemon Pancakes
2 teaspoons margarine or butter
1 cup 1% low-fat milk

LUNCH *Snappy Seafood Salad
1 whole wheat pita pocket
1 pear

DINNER *Stuffed Bell Peppers
*Green Salad
1 whole grain roll
1 teaspoon margarine or butter
*Apple Cake
1 cup 1% low-fat milk

Day 14 1865 calories
50 grams of fat (24% of calories)
28 grams of fiber

BREAKFAST *1 slice Blueberry Orange Bread
*Berry Banana Smoothie

LUNCH   *Tomato Basil Soup
2 ounces boiled ham
1 ounce cheese (preferably a lower-fat cheese)
2 slices whole grain bread
mustard

DINNER   *Chicken Breasts in Creamy Mustard Sauce
*Dilly Carrots
1 cup noodles, preferably whole wheat
2 plums
*Apple Cake (leftover from Day 13)
1 cup 1% low-fat milk

Part Five

===

The Principles Behind the Self-Help
Nutritional Program

18   *Increasing Fiber*

*I*n the 1950s, D. P. Burkett, the British surgeon and epidemiologist, observed that low-fiber diets seemed to be associated with an increased incidence of appendicitis, colon cancer, diverticulosis, and hiatal hernia. He went to Africa to study populations where these ailments were almost unknown, and compared their diet with the British diet. At the same time, he methodically collected, measured, and compared stool specimens from both populations. He found that the typical Englishman produced 200 grams of stool a day, while the African tribesman produced over 600 grams a day. The reason, Burkett concluded was that the Africans consumed large quantities of natural fiber in the form of whole grains, seeds, and nuts, while the English consumed very little.

A low-fiber diet is also low in residue, causing food wastes to pass slowly through the bowel, with serious consequences. Irritable bowel syndrome, diverticulitis, diverticular bleeding and perforation are all associated with low-residue diets. Cancer of the colon has also been linked to low-fiber diets because there is more time for carcinogens present in the stool to come in contact with the gut wall.

Positive Effects of Fiber

Conversely, high-fiber diets increase the bulk in stool and cause it to pass through the bowel more quickly. High-fiber foods also absorb toxins and prevent pollutants from being absorbed into the body. In one animal study, rats were fed either a low-fiber diet or a high-fiber diet along with a variety of possibly harmful food additives and/or toxic chemicals. The rats that ate a high-fiber diet lived longer and in better health, despite the addition of toxins, than those fed a low-fiber diet.

In another unusual animal study, researchers fed rats small amounts of three potentially harmful food additives. None were harmed when given individual food additives. With two additives in the diet, however, the animals experienced various symptoms, including balding, scruffy fur, diarrhea, and poor weight gain. When another group of animals were fed all three food additives at once, they all died within two weeks. Yet when a control group of animals were fed all three additives *plus* a high-fiber diet, all survived unharmed.

The latest news on the benefits of high-fiber diets is from a recently completed long-term study at Memorial Sloan-Kettering Center and Cornell University—New York Hospital. Over a period of four years, researchers found that high-fiber diets inhibited the growth of rectal polyps, which can lead to cancer, in people with an inherited tendency toward such polyps.

A diet high in fiber is now recommended by the National Cancer Institute, the Food and Nutrition Board, and the National Academy of Sciences.

Fiber is a near miraculous protector of the intestinal tract and improves GI problems across the board.

- Fiber relieves constipation by making the stool bulkier and softer.

- Fiber stops diarrhea by absorbing excess water in the stool. For the same reason, it helps mild cases of colitis.

- Fiber helps relieve hemorrhoids, diverticulosis discomfort, and IBS.

- Fiber provides some protection against the formation of gallstones and development of colon cancer.

- Fiber can help heal and prevent ulcers.

- A high-fiber diet helps control weight, reduce blood cholesterol, and control blood sugar levels.

What Kind of Fiber

Fiber is material from plant cell walls that resists digestion and is largely excreted in the stool. Some fiber ferments in the digestive tract, producing small-chain fatty acids, the major nutrient for the colon.

There are two main categories of fiber: water insoluble and water soluble. Both kinds are found in the same foods, but the ratio varies. We've only recently realized that different fibers have different effects.

• Insoluble Fiber

Insoluble fiber primarily increases stool bulk and water content, speeding transit of stool through the bowel. Because it is a natural laxative, insoluble fiber is effective in preventing diverticulitis and treating irritable bowel syndrome and hemorrhoids. Insoluble fiber is also believed to lessen the risk of colon cancer, possibly by reducing the amount of time carcinogens remain in the GI system. Some insoluble fibers also decrease the amount of bile acids in the stomach, which makes them an ideal treatment for ulcers. Wheat bran is the most concentrated form of insoluble fiber, but all whole grains and many fruits and vegetables also contain large quantities.

• Soluble Fiber

Soluble fiber absorbs water and slows down food transit from the stomach. The greatest benefit of soluble fiber is that it helps decrease cholesterol levels in your blood by washing bile acids from the intestinal tract. Because it gives a feeling of fullness for a longer period of time, soluble fiber controls appetite and enhances weight-loss diets, even in obese people. Soluble fiber also helps protect against both hypoglycemia and hyperglycemia because it helps your system maintain an even level of blood sugar. Dried beans, whole oats, and oat bran are the most concentrated forms of soluble fiber. (Dried beans and legumes may cause gas, however. See Chapter 22 for tips on how to reduce gas.)

Insoluble Fibers	Soluble Fibers
Wheat bran	Oat bran
Corn bran	Whole oats
Whole grains	Rice bran
Dried beans and peas	Dried beans
Popcorn	Chick peas, black-eyed peas
Seeds and nuts	Lentils
Most fruit and vegetables, especially carrots, white potatoes, sweet potatoes, artichokes, broccoli, leeks, parsnips	Sesame seeds
	All fruits and vegetables, especially citrus fruits, apples, pears, sweet potatoes, carrots, okra, cauliflower, corn

Using Fiber to Help GI Disorders

The goal of the Self-Help Nutritional Program is to change your diet to include more foods naturally high in fiber. Fiber is found in carbohydrates—grains and cereals, fruits and vegetables. Carbohydrates may be either simple or complex. Complex carbohydrates require quite a bit of processing by the digestive tract to break them down into absorbable nutrients. Grains and cereals fall into this category, and this is the kind of complex carbohydrates your muscular GI system likes best. Fruits and vegetables, which have more sugars, also contain complex carbohydrates and are also good sources of fiber.

Because different fibers have different beneficial effects, the Self-Help Nutritional Program recommends using a wide variety of complex carbohydrates daily—whole grains, cereals, fresh fruits and vegetables. Such a wide range of ingredients also adds color and interest to recipes, and helps keep you feeling satisfied. Deriving fiber from several different sources also prevents the gassiness and abdominal discomfort sometimes associated with wheat bran alone.

• About Bran

Bran, the outer shell of wheat, oats, rice, and other whole grains, is the most concentrated form of both soluble and insoluble fiber. The natural fibers found inside fruits, vegetables, and grains have exactly the same benefits attributed to bran, although in a less concentrated form. Obviously, bran is present in all whole grains. Various brans can also be purchased separately.

When you consume a diet that emphasizes fiber-rich foods across the board there is no need to consume additional quantities of bran. A bowl of cooked oat bran cereal is fine if you like it, but a bowl of oatmeal is every bit as good. You may also add bran to your own recipe creations if you wish, but the recipes in this program are designed to provide substantial amounts of fiber, and it's unnecessary to add wheat bran or oat bran to recipes and foods that are already naturally fiber-filled.

If you do choose to add bran to your recipes, however, it's important to remember that soluble bran such as oat bran seems to work best when it's cooked. Insoluble bran, such as wheat bran, tends to be more effective when it is uncooked. Coarsely ground wheat bran also appears to work better than finely ground bran, even though the two are chemically identical.

• Vegetables against Free Radicals

Vegetables are an excellent source of fiber. Eating vegetables of all kinds on a regular basis helps a wide range of GI problems, and also plays a vital role in preventing other diseases. For instance, beta-carotene and other carotenoids—pigments found in many yellow, orange, and red vegetables and dark green leafy vegetables (beet greens, broccoli, carrots, spinach)—help combat cancers of the mouth, throat, lung, stomach, and bladder, and possibly cancer of the colon and cervix. These disease-fighting carotenoids are thought to protect healthy cells of the body against damage by molecules known as free radicals, which are found in air pollution and food additives.

In the body, free radicals cause a chemical reaction (oxidation) that can produce disease by changing the structure of cells. Carotenoids are *antioxidants*—they destroy free radicals before they can do harm. Because we are exposed to free radicals every day, we need to eat plenty of carotenoid-rich vegetables like broccoli and carrots. Vegetables rich in vitamins C and E, such as asparagus, cabbage, and sweet potatoes, are also potent antioxidants and may fight many types of cancer.

A few of these cancer-fighting vegetables, particularly cabbage, are known to aggravate some GI disorders. You will notice that the Two-Week Master Program uses asparagus and sweet potatoes to supply antioxidants, but avoids cabbage. Check your Flag Foods carefully and experiment with vegetables. Fortunately, there are many carotenoid-rich vegetables that the GI tract likes.

Drinking More Water

Most people don't think of water as food, but all of us need a certain amount of water to maintain life. About half of the human body is made of water. Every single cell needs water to maintain itself. Much of our water is in foods; we also consume large amounts of water in the form of coffee, tea, soft drinks, milk, and other liquids.

Since fiber absorbs considerable amounts of water, it is important that you drink plenty of water with the Self-Help Nutritional Program. You need about 30 cubic centimeters of water per kilogram of body weight every day, or 1 cc for every calorie that you consume. Therefore, if you consume an average of 2000 calories a day, you need 2000 cc of fluid each day—or eight 8-ounce glasses of water. (By the way, drinking water will not increase your body's fluid retention. And it won't make you feel heavy and bloated.)

19   *Lowering Fat*

*F*ats have many jobs to perform in the body: small quantities are used for body repair and growth of tissues; fat also provides fatty tissues for insulation and is essential to the body's use of certain vitamins. Fats also provide energy.

Too much fat, however, causes problems for the digestive tract. Fat makes the gallbladder work hard, which is a problem if you have gallstones or gallbladder disease. It relaxes the LES valve, which lets stomach acids back up into the esophagus. Fat also stimulates the pancreas, which can cause pain if you have pancreatitis. High-fat diets are associated with increased risk of many chronic diseases, including cancer and heart disease.

Fat is also by far the most concentrated source of calories, with more than twice as many calories per gram as protein or carbohydrate. Studies on overweight people show that the degree of obesity has more to do with the percentage of fat intake than with surplus calories from all sources. Furthermore, fat calories are stored more efficiently than carbohydrate or protein calories, which makes it easy for the body to convert dietary fat into body fat, and very hard for the body to convert carbohydrates into fat.

Help for GI Problems

Reducing fat in the diet relieves heartburn, prevents gallbladder attacks, and aids pancreatitis. A low-fat diet also helps prevent colon cancer and the development of kidney stones in people with Crohn's disease. Reducing *total* fat helps control weight and also helps prevent other diseases associated with high-fat diets such as heart disease and certain cancers, including breast cancer.

The primary goal of the Self-Help Nutritional Program is to decrease the *total fat* in your diet. In the Two-Week Master Program, all kinds of fats are minimized. The program supplies only 21 to 28 per-

How Many Grams of Fat?

The goal is to derive less than 30 percent of your daily calories from fat. To discover how much fat you can eat each day and stay within the guideline, do this simple calculation:

1. Multiply your daily calories by .3
2. Divide the result by 9, the number of calories in each gram of fat

The result is the total number of grams of fat you can eat per day. Only one-third of this total should come from saturated fat (described further below). Following are some examples.

Calories per Day	Grams of Fat per Day	Grams of Saturated Fat per Day
1200	40 or less	13 or less
1500	50 or less	17 or less
1800	60 or less	20 or less
2100	70 or less	23 or less
2400	80 or less	27 or less

How Much Is a Gram?*

Many packaged food products offer nutritional information, including number of grams of fat. For quick reference, there are 5 grams of fat in each of the following:

1 teaspoon of oil, margarine, mayonnaise, or butter

1 tablespoon of regular salad dressings, diet margarine, or diet mayonnaise

1 tablespoon of cashews

5 large olives

10 large peanuts

⅛ avocado

2 whole walnuts or pecans

6 whole almonds

* Adapted from the American Dietetic Association and the American Diabetic Association Exchange List for Meal Planning

cent of calories from fat each day, even less than the amount recommended by the National Cancer Institute. Your lifelong objective is to maintain this low consumption.

It is much easier to monitor your fat intake by counting grams than by calculating percentages. The box opposite gives you a quick way to keep track of your daily fat intake.

Fats can be reduced by decreasing the amount, eliminating the fat, or employing cooking methods that do not require fat. The fats used in the Master Program are usually from vegetable oils; if a recipe calls for a saturated fat such as butter, a very small amount is used.

Good Fats vs. Bad Fats

All fats are high in calories and used slowly by the body; however, some fats are more deleterious than others.

Fats are either saturated or unsaturated. Saturated fats can elevate blood cholesterol; unsaturated fats do not increase blood cholesterol. For the most part, saturated fats are derived from animal foods —meat, milk, and butter; unsaturated fats are found in vegetable oils. There are a few critical exceptions.

• Polyunsaturated Vegetable Oils

For more than two decades polyunsaturated vegetable oils have been recognized as heart-healthy alternatives to butter and other fats derived from animal products. But new research indicates that what might be good for the heart is bad for the immune system. Polyunsaturated oils are high in omega-6 fatty acids. New findings from animal studies show that diets high in omega-6 stimulated the growth of tumors of the breast, pancreas, and colon.

• Tropical Vegetable Oils

Vegetable oils derived from coconut, palm, and palm kernel are highly saturated. Nondairy creamers, cookies, and other baked products and snack foods are typical products that contain tropical oils. Food companies have recently been under pressure to remove highly saturated tropical oils from processed foods. Tropical oils are often replaced with partially hydrogenated oils that contain trans fatty acids. New studies suggest that these trans fats may be just as harmful as saturated fat and tropical oils.

• Margarine and Solid Shortenings

Trans fatty acids are produced when liquid vegetable oil is hardened, or hydrogenated, to produce margarine or solid vegetable shortening. When vegetable oil is hydrogenated, some fatty acids become more saturated, while others are changed into trans fatty acids. Researchers believe that these trans fatty acids act like saturated fats to lower the good form of cholesterol—high-density lipoprotein, or HDL—that protects against heart disease, while increasing the level of harmful cholesterol—low-density lipoprotein, or LDL.

Any processed food that contains partially hydrogenated oil contains trans fats: crackers, cookies, pastries, cakes, doughnuts, french fries, potato chips, puddings, and graham crackers.

Some researchers believe that trans fatty acids should be counted as saturated fats. Under current labeling rules, if specific fat information is provided on a food label, trans fats are included among the more healthful monounsaturated fats. (Most of the fatty acids that are converted to trans fatty acids during hydrogenation are monounsaturated fats.) Under normal conditions monounsaturated fats are generally thought to protect against heart disease.

Other researchers believe that trans fats are not harmful, unless consumed in large quantities. By following a program that limits fat intake to less than 30 percent of calories, the intake of trans fats, as well as saturated fats and cholesterol, is automatically reduced.

If you use margarine, choose tub margarine, which is lower in both saturated and trans fatty acids. (Stick margarine generally has twice as much fatty acids as softer tub margarines.) Margarines or spreads that list liquid oil as the first ingredient are a better choice than those that list partially hydrogenated oil first. Liquid squeeze margarines are the lowest in saturated and trans fats. Liquid oils and foods like corn oil or mayonnaise that list liquid oils as the first ingredient are also low in saturated and trans fats.

• Olive and Canola Oil: Monounsaturates

Monounsaturated fat has become the "fat of choice." Like the polyunsaturates, monounsaturates lower *total* cholesterol. They may do even more to protect your heart, however, because they are more selective when they go to work on cholesterol. Cholesterol is broken into several different factors. Generally, HDLs are good factors, working to keep arteries clean; LDLs cause the artery-clogging damage. Monounsaturated fats lower total cholesterol without lowering the good HDLs. Not all monounsaturates have this effect, however.

Olive oil is a good choice for cooking because it is one of the richest sources of monounsaturated fat in the diet. More than three-quarters of its fat is monounsaturated, virtually none of it in the trans form. Canola oil (rapeseed oil), sold in supermarkets under the Puritan label, is almost as high in monounsaturated fat but is lower in saturated fat than olive oil.

Peanut oil and avocado oil, although monounsaturates, are saturated to the extent that they provide a neutral effect. They are not harmful, but don't provide the same benefit as olive oil or canola oil.

• Omega-3 Fatty Acids

Omega-3 fatty acids, found in fish oils, benefit the body in several ways. They have the reverse effect of omega-6, slowing tumor growth. Omega-3 fatty acids are also heart-healthy. Early observations in Greenland showed that Eskimos, despite a diet high in fat and cholesterol, had a low incidence of heart disease. Closer examination showed that while their total cholesterol was high, their triglycerides, another blood fat linked to heart disease, were low. The Eskimos also had high HDLs, the good cholesterol. This good ratio of cholesterol factors was traced to the high proportion of omega-3 fatty acids in the traditional Eskimo diet of fish and other marine animals.

Omega-3 fatty acids also reduce clotting of the blood, which helps prevent the progression of coronary artery disease. Certain fishes are high in omega-3 fatty acids, especially salmon, tuna, mackerel, herring, sardines, halibut, and trout.

Recommendations for the Self-Help Nutritional Program

More research is needed before specific recommendations for desirable amounts of polyunsaturates, monounsaturates, or fish oils can be given.

The most important point is to reduce total fat intake by using fats from all sources sparingly. Only one-third of your total fat intake should come from saturated fats; the balance should come from monounsaturated and/or polyunsaturated fats. The Two-Week Master Program, which supplies 21 to 28 percent of calories from fats each day, automatically does this for you.

• Fat and Heart Disease

The major risk factors for heart disease are high blood pressure, cigarette smoking, obesity, and high blood cholesterol. Dietary fat, especially animal fat, increases the level of cholesterol in your blood. Certain lower-fat foods can also boost cholesterol in the blood, even though they tend to have less impact than dietary fat: egg yolks, organ meats such as liver and kidney, caviar, fish roe, and shellfish all contain large quantities of cholesterol.

Cholesterol is a natural fatty substance manufactured in the liver and also present in many foods that we eat. When the body doesn't burn all its fats, cholesterol is laid down like silt along the inside of the arteries where it forms a hard pastelike deposit, which narrows the arteries and as a result increases your risk of heart disease and premature death

About 25 percent of Americans between the ages of 20 and 74 have high blood cholesterol, which translates into at least 40 million people. Anyone at any age can have high blood cholesterol. For unknown reasons, not everyone who eats a high-fat diet has elevated cholesterol, and some people who eat an exceedingly low-fat diet do have elevated blood cholesterol. The answer to this mysterious paradox may lie in genetics: some people use cholesterol more efficiently than others. It's also an interesting fact that cholesterol levels tend to jump when you are under stress.

One thing we know for sure: many people can lower their blood cholesterol levels by making alterations in their diet. These include reducing fat and increasing fiber, particularly soluble fiber (in the form of oat bran, whole oats, and dried beans), which acts like a sponge to mop up excess cholesterol and transport it out of the bloodstream.

A federal advisory panel has labeled total blood cholesterol above 240 milligrams per deciliter of blood as high blood cholesterol, 200 to 239 as borderline, and below 200 as desirable. The panel advises everyone over age 20 to have total cholesterol measured at least once every five years, and those classified borderline to have the test repeated. There is new evidence that even children can have elevated cholesterol, which can lead to problems later in life. At this time, children probably do not need to have their cholesterol checked routinely unless there is a strong history of high cholesterol and early heart attack in the family.

Cholesterol-lowering drugs are now available, but are usually recommended only for those with the highest risk of heart disease or when changes in diet fail to do the job.

Which Fats Are Which?

Monounsaturated	Polyunsaturated	Saturated
Olive oil	Safflower oil	Butter
Canola oil	Sunflower oil	Meat fat
Peanut oil	Corn oil	Lard (pork fat)
Avocados	Soybean oil	Hydrogenated fats§
Olives	Cottonseed oil	Cream
Peanuts	Margarines†	Cheese
Peanut butter*	Sesame oil	Whole milk
Cashews	Mayonnaise	Coconut oil
Almonds	Walnuts	Palm kernel oil
Pecans	Fish oils‡	Palm oil

* Peanut butter that is natural, ground from pure peanuts, contains monounsaturated fat. Peanut butter that has been hydrogenated has been processed in a way that makes its fats more saturated. Most commercially made peanut butters available at your supermarket are hydrogenated. In natural peanut butters the oil rises to the top; to decrease total fat content, pour off oil before using.

† Margarines differ in their ratio of saturated to unsaturated fat. Generally, the softer the margarine, the higher the polyunsaturates. If the first ingredient listed on the label is a hydrogenated vegetable oil, then the product is higher in saturated fat. Look for a liquid oil as the first ingredient on the margarine label. Ingredients on all labels are listed in order of decreasing predominance.

‡ Fish oils are high in the omega-3 fatty acids that fight cholesterol.

§ Hydrogenated fats are polyunsaturated fats that have been processed to make them solid. The processing also makes them saturated.

• Fat and Cancer

The role of fat in cancer is not yet well documented, but it appears that high-fat diets may stimulate the production of substances that increase the risk of various cancers. For example, dietary fat stimulates the production and release of bile acids from the liver and gallbladder. These acids are then more readily converted to a carcinogen, or cancer-causing substance. Bile acids may also injure healthy tissue in the colon. Both mechanisms may play a role in increasing the risk of colon cancer. Dietary fat may also stimulate hormones that promote tumor growth. Thus, high-fat diets have been associated with an increased risk of cancer of the breast and endometrium in women, the prostate in men, and the colon in both men and women.

To reduce the risk of heart disease and cancer, the National Cancer Institute has advised Americans to reduce their intake of fat from all sources to less than 30 percent of total daily calories. According to the National Cancer Institute, not everything you eat needs to be less than 30 percent fat. The 30 percent figure is for the entire day. Therefore, if you eat an ice cream cone that is 80 percent fat, you can balance it against a dish with much less fat. For people with GI disorders, however, it is much better to avoid high-fat foods across the board, because a single serving of high-fat food can act as a trigger on the GI tract.

Avoid Cholesterol-Packed Foods

Many foods that raise blood cholesterol also have a negative effect on the GI tract. You can do double duty—protect your arteries and soothe your digestive disorder—if you avoid or use sparingly foods that promote cholesterol in the blood:

Beef—ground chuck, short ribs, processed meats such as corned beef, salami, sausage, bologna, frankfurters

Veal—all cuts, especially the breast

Lamb—chops and ribs

Pork—shoulder, loin, sausage, chitterlings, spareribs, salami

All fried foods

Whole-milk dairy products, cheeses with more than 5 grams of fat per ounce, ice cream, cream, butter

Nondairy creamers

Processed foods—especially those that contain coconut oil, palm kernel or palm oil, animal fat, or hydrogenated oils

Sauces such as hollandaise and béarnaise, quiche lorraine

Egg yolks—limit yourself to three or four a week, or substitute egg whites for whole eggs in recipes

20 Reducing Lactose

A low-lactose diet helps those who suffer from intestinal gas and lactose intolerance, one of the world's most common GI complaints (see Chapter 10). The gas and diarrhea resulting from "milk" intolerance is caused by the milk sugar lactose, and not the milk itself or its fat content. Skim milk will cause as much trouble in lactose-intolerant people as whole milk with regard to GI symptoms.

Lactose is found in all dairy products, which are also a major source of calcium and other beneficial nutrients. Fortunately, it isn't necessary to abandon dairy products on the Self-Help Nutritional Program, even if you are lactose intolerant. There are several alternatives to regular dairy products that can be used by those who are lactose intolerant.

Acidophilus Milk

Acidophilus milk is regular milk with the active lactobacillus added to it. This bacterial culture has the ability to make lactase, the enzyme that allows us to digest lactose. Warmed in your digestive system, acidophilus starts to work to break down lactose.

This milk cannot be used in cooking or added to a hot drink, because heat kills the lactobacillus. If you choose acidophilus milk, use it for drinking. Acidophilus milk is available at your supermarket or health food store. It tastes the same as regular milk.

Lactaid Milk

Ready-made milk called Lactaid comes with lactase, the enzyme that digests lactose, already in it. You can buy 1% low-fat or skim Lactaid milk in your supermarket.

Lactaid milk tends to stay fresher and taste sweeter than regular milk because the enzyme has pre-split the milk sugar lactose into sweeter-tasting glucose and galactose. Because this milk is predigested, it is heat stable—you can heat it and it will still help symptoms of lactose intolerance. However, Lactaid milk usually breaks down only about 70 percent of the lactose in milk. Most people can handle the remaining 30 percent. Some people, however, are so lactose intolerant that they require milk products that are 100-percent lactose-free.

Lactase Enzyme: Drops and Tablets

For those who are highly sensitive to lactose and require 100-percent conversion, the lactase enzyme itself can be added to milk products. The addition of lactase enzyme gives the milk a sweet taste, although the milk actually contains no more carbohydrates or calories than regular milk.

The lactase enzyme is available as a liquid that can be added to milk or in a tablet form that can be taken when you ingest milk products. Both are sold under various brand names at your health food store or pharmacy.

Instructions for the lactose enzyme liquid are given on the package label, but you will probably need to use more than the recommended amount to make the milk as close to 100-percent lactose-free as possible. After adding the drops to milk, allow the mixture to sit in the refrigerator for twenty-four hours before using it. You may then use the lactose-free milk for drinking or in any recipe that calls for milk.

Instead of treating the milk with drops, you can treat your digestive tract with lactase enzyme tablets. Take one or two tablets whenever you drink untreated milk or eat cheese, ice cream, or any products or dishes made with dairy products.

Fermented Milk Products

Even people who are lactose intolerant can usually tolerate small amounts of lactose. Fermented or processed milk products such as yogurt, butter, hard and soft ripened cheeses, buttermilk, and sour cream usually do not cause digestive problems. In these products the lactobacilli have predigested some of the lactose. Yogurt that contains live cultures is even easier to digest. (Yogurt that isn't made with live cultures will probably have the same effect as milk.)

Adjusting Lactose in Your Diet

For those who suffer from gas, we recommend that when first starting the Two-Week Master Program you purchase lactase enzyme liquid or tablets. (All of the recipes in the recipe section indicate how many lactase enzyme tablets to take with the meal.)

You can begin to discover your personal tolerance level by gradually adding small amounts of regular milk products to your diet, while observing for symptoms of flatulence, diarrhea, or abdominal cramps. Try using regular milk in your coffee, or experimenting with fermented milk products such as yogurt and cheese. If no symptoms occur, begin to use regular milk products in your recipes.

21 *Lowering Spice Content*

Spicy foods may stimulate acid secretion and cause sudden spasms of the esophagus in certain people predisposed to spasms. Spices may also aggravate preexisting digestive disorders, such as esophagitis and IBS, and exacerbate their symptoms.

Documentation of the negative effects of specific spices on the GI tract are scarce, however. One study that tracked the effect of spices in the diets of ulcer patients showed that the spices most strongly linked to gastric distress are black pepper, chili pepper, mustard seed, cloves, and nutmeg. Symptoms are generally worse if spicy foods are eaten on an empty stomach. Garlic, chili, and curry powder are also irritating spices for many people with GI complaints.

Not all spices are irritating to the stomach. Those least likely to exert a harmful effect are cinnamon, allspice, mace, thyme, sage, paprika, and caraway seed.

Overall, a low-spice regimen can be expected to benefit heartburn, ulcers, and IBS. Most of the recipes in the Self-Help Nutritional Program have been developed without spices. If you are able to tolerate spices, use your imagination and add them whenever you wish. Herbs such as thyme, rosemary, basil, sage, and others may be added to, or substituted in, recipes to suit your own taste.

Effect of Spices on the GI Tract

Most Aggravating	*Least Aggravating*
Black pepper	Allspice
Chili pepper	Caraway seed
Chili powder	Cinnamon
Cloves	Mace
Curry powder	Paprika
Garlic	Sage
Mustard seed	Thyme
Nutmeg	

22   *Reducing Gas-Forming Legumes*

The process of digestion always produces gas, but some people—especially people with GI disorders—may react adversely to even small amounts of gas in the GI tract. For example, even a little excessive gas for someone who suffers from IBS can produce spasm and pain. People with certain conditions or diseases—previous surgery on the GI tract, very low secretion of stomach acid, immune deficiency disorders, strictures of the small intestine, longstanding diabetes—may develop an overgrowth of bacteria in parts of the GI tract usually devoid of bacteria; these pockets of extra bacteria digest carbohydrates and produce excessive quantities of gas. Some healthy people also produce excessive quantities of gas simply because of the type of bacteria present in their GI tract.

We know that certain foods create more gas than others, and that reducing these gas-forming foods in the diet can help improve certain GI conditions. Unfortunately, many of the worst offenders are also good for you. Beans, for example, are nourishing, inexpensive, and so versatile that they are used in every kind of cuisine. They are also major producers of flatus because their carbohydrates are so difficult to digest that gas-producing bacteria in the colon have a field day. The disease-fighting cruciferous vegetables, which include the cabbage family, also tend to be gas producers. If you suffer from excessive gas you'll need to experiment with foods. Each person is different, and there is no need to eliminate foods that don't bother you.

Some people can reduce excessive gas simply by making the above changes. I had one patient who began suffering from excessive gas seemingly without cause. Lisa had never complained of gas before, but on a routine visit told me that she had noticed that she was always "gassy" and it was starting to bother her. I showed Lisa the list below, and she checked seven out of nine items. She was surprised, and so was I. The only two risk factors she *didn't have* were constipation and air swallowing. Lisa had recently been under a lot of stress and had fallen into poor eating habits, a combination of factors that produced excessive gas. She gulped her meals, overate once or twice a day,

---

Steps to Reduce Excessive Gas

Many people find that if they eat legumes and cruciferous vegetables several times a week in small quantities, gas production subsides. You can also reduce the gas production of beans by changing the way you prepare them. Cook dried beans using the quick-soak method: Bring dried beans to a boil for 2 minutes, then turn off heat and let stand for 1 hour. Drain water. Add fresh water, then cook beans as usual. This cooking method reduces gas production by about 20 percent.

Another way to help the bowel digest these gas-forming foods is to add yogurt with active cultures to your diet. Yogurt bacteria help digest these foods and slow down gas production.

Here are some further steps you can take to prevent the occurrence of excessive gas.

1. Eat slowly.
2. Chew your food well.
3. Avoid eating when you feel tense or upset.
4. Don't overload your stomach. Keep meal sizes moderate.
5. Limit fluids with meals.
6. Avoid constipation.
7. Limit carbonated beverages.
8. Exercise.
9. Eliminate gum chewing, smoking, sucking on hard candies, drinking through straws or from bottles, and gulping large quantities of fluid. All these activities encourage air swallowing.

---

drank quantities of club soda, and used food to calm her anxiety. She got almost no exercise. Lisa didn't have to change the types of food she ate, but she did have to change the way she ate them. This proved to be a simple adjustment for her to make.

The strategy we used to create recipes for the Self-Help Nutritional Program was to avoid beans altogether, and use very few legumes. This was accomplished for the most part by substituting whole grains, such as bulgur wheat and kasha, and other vegetables for beans and legumes. Some foods such as broccoli, known to be gas-forming, are used in the recipes for the Two-Week Master Program. However, these foods are marked as Flag Foods, and a substitute such as carrots is offered for people who have trouble with gas.

Beano, a new product from the makers of Lactaid, contains the enzyme α-galactosidase, which aids in the digestion of beans and legumes. It can be purchased OTC at your pharmacy.

23 *Low Calories/High Nutrition*

*O*ne of the most important goals of the Self-Help Nutritional Program is to control your calorie intake so that you maintain a desirable body weight. Overeating and excess weight can have a devastating effect on GI disorders, including heartburn and gallstones.

Problems Associated with Being Overweight

Extra weight in the abdomen increases pressure under the LES valve, the one-way valve located between the esophagus and the stomach, and causes acid to back up. Clothes that fit tightly around the waist also increase pressure on the abdomen, which in turn builds up the pressure under the LES. People who are overweight often wear clothes that are too tight because of recent weight gain, or the wishful notion that if they buy the same size as they always have they haven't really gained weight. But even if your clothes are a perfect fit, you are still more likely to have heartburn if you are overweight. Fat isn't deposited only under the skin where you can feel it and see it, it is also deposited deep within the body. Fat accumulates around internal organs, especially around the intestines and the abdominal lining. As fat fills up the interior of the abdomen, pressure builds up under the LES, causing reflux. Losing weight may not be as easy as chewing antacid tablets, but it's a much more effective and long-lasting way to treat heartburn.

Intestinal gas and flatulence are also common GI responses to excess weight. People who overeat, especially if they eat large quantities of food in one sitting, produce excessive gas. Overeating can also cause distress if you have IBS.

Belching is another by-product of excess weight. The more you weigh, the more difficult it is to exercise; the less exercise you do, the more weight you gain. When you do exert yourself, there is a lot of huffing and puffing, and you tend to swallow more air than usual. Just as extra weight in the abdomen causes stomach acid to back up into the esophagus, it also causes excess air to back up. Losing weight encourages you to be more active, makes breathing easier, and belching usually subsides.

When you are overweight fat may also infiltrate vital organs, although fatty infiltration doesn't cause specific GI problems for most people. Severely obese people may lose some function of the pancreas. Since the pancreas normally produces far more enzymes than are necessary to digest food, however, some loss of function usually doesn't pose any problem. Even people who have had most of the pancreas surgically removed because of chronic pancreatitis or cancer still have normal digestive function.

Fatty infiltration of the liver, however, is another story. Like the pancreas, the liver usually continues to function normally up to a point because there is a tremendous reserve of function. Occasionally, however, a fatty liver becomes inflamed, a process called steatohepatitis, which sets up a potentially dangerous condition. Inflammation can lead to scarring and, in some cases, cirrhosis. The worst part is that liver inflammation may not produce any noticeable symptoms. The surest cure is prevention by losing weight before the condition develops. (Once scarring has occurred, the damage is irreversible.)

Obesity is strongly associated with gallstones. The liver manufactures bile, which is then stored in the gallbladder and released as needed to digest fats. Bile is mainly composed of bile salts, phospholipids, and cholesterol. When you are overweight, bile becomes supersaturated with cholesterol. Stored in the gallbladder, the cholesterol-rich bile begins to crystallize and the particles join together to form a stone. Stones can cause serious problems if they migrate out of the gallbladder and get stuck in the bile ducts.

Maintaining ideal weight definitely prevents the formation of gallstones. In a recent study published in the *New England Journal of Medicine,* investigators at Harvard University reported a one-to-one correlation between weight and risk for gallstones. The more you weigh, the higher the risk. But surprisingly, *losing* weight may increase the risk of getting stones. Prolonged fasting or modified fasting as part of a rapid weight-loss program causes the gallbladder to become inactive because very little fat (1–2 grams per day) is being processed. Bile that would normally be ejected to help digest fats stagnates in the gallbladder, becomes more saturated with cholesterol, and makes stone formation more likely.

Excess weight is also associated with other medical conditions—heart disease; adult onset diabetes mellitus; high blood pressure; cancer of the breast, endometrium, and prostate; cancer of the colon and rectum; arthritis of the knees and hips; varicose veins; gout; and respiratory problems.

Self-Help

The Self-Help Nutritional Program is a naturally low-calorie program because it reduces fat calories. It also increases carbohydrates and controls the amount of protein you consume. Many people believe that a low-calorie diet should emphasize protein to guarantee nutritional health. They believe that a high-fiber, low-calorie combination will leave out essential nutrients. The secret lies in getting maximum nutrition from minimal calories.

• Proteins and Carbohydrates

Proteins are the compounds that form the basic structure of all living matter. A regular daily intake of protein helps all body cells and tissues repair and replace themselves and grow. Protein is important for making hormones and enzymes, and for proper immune function.

There are two kinds of protein: animal-derived proteins (meat, fish, eggs, and dairy products) and vegetable proteins (peas, beans and other legumes, and grains). Animal protein is often called high-quality protein because it is made in precisely the form the body requires. However, animal protein is inevitably accompanied by high quantities of fats. Vegetable proteins, on the other hand, when combined, can add up to valuable protein without the excess fat.

Some people think that protein is less fattening than starchy carbohydrates. This isn't true: gram for gram, protein and carbohydrate contain the same amount of calories. But because animal protein is dense, it doesn't take much volume to add up to a lot of calories and it's easy to eat more protein than you actually need at any one time. If you eat more protein than you require for replacement of body tissues, the excess is used to provide extra energy or is stored in the body as fat.

• How Much Protein?

The average American consumes about 100 grams of protein daily, almost twice as much as most adults need. Depending on your size, you need only 50 to 80 grams of protein a day to maintain good health.

Protein needs are calculated at .8 grams per kilogram (2.2 pounds) of body weight per day. So if you weigh 130 pounds you need less than 50 grams of protein a day.

You will obtain 7 grams of protein from each ounce of meat, fish,

Grams of Protein in Common Foods

Food	Serving Size	Grams of Protein
Barley	¼ cup raw	4.1
Bean curd (tofu)	1 piece (4 ounces)	9.4
Beans, kidney	½ cup cooked	7.2
Beans, lima	½ cup cooked	6.5
Beans, navy	½ cup cooked	7.4
Bean sprouts, mung	½ cup, raw or cooked	2.0
Beef, lean ground	¼ pound raw	23.4
Bran flakes (40%)	1 cup	3.6
Bread, white	1 slice	2.4
Bread, whole wheat	1 slice	2.6
Broccoli	1 cup cooked	8.4
Bulgur	1 cup cooked	2.7
Cheese, American	1 ounce	6.6
Cheese, cheddar	1 ounce	7.1
Cheese, cottage	½ cup	15.0
Chicken	1 drumstick	12.2
Corn	½ cup kernels	3.2
Eggs	2 medium	11.4
Farina	½ cup cooked in water	3.2
Flounder	3 ounces	25.5
Frankfurter	1 (2 ounces)	7.1
Ham, boiled	3 slices (3 ounces)	16.2
Lamb, rib chop	3 ounces	17.9
Lentils	½ cup cooked	7.8
Liver, chicken	1 liver	6.6
Macaroni	1 cup cooked	6.5
Mackerel	3 ounces	17.9

Food	Serving Size	Grams of Protein
Milk, skim	1 cup	8.8
Noodles, egg	1 cup cooked	6.6
Oatmeal	1 cup cooked in water	4.8
Pancakes	3 4-inch cakes	5.7
Peanut butter	2 tablespoons	8.0
Peas, green	½ cup cooked	4.3
Pork, loin	3 ounces	20.8
Pork sausage	2 links (2 ounces)	5.4
Potato	7 ounces baked	4.0
Rice, brown	1 cup cooked	4.9
Rice, white	1 cup cooked	4.1
Scallops	3 ounces	16.0
Sesame seeds	1 tablespoon	1.5
Shrimp	3 ounces	11.6
Soup, bean with pork	1 cup, made with water	8.0
Soup, tomato	1 cup, made with milk	6.5
Soybeans	½ cup cooked	9.9
Spaghetti	1 cup cooked al dente	6.5
Squash, acorn	1 cup baked	3.9
Sweet potato	5 ounces baked	2.4
Tuna, canned	3 ounces, drained	24.4
Turkey	3 ounces	26.8
Veal, stew meat	3 ounces	23.7
Walnuts	10 large	7.3
Wheat flakes	1 cup	3.1
Wheat, shredded	1 cup	5.0
Yogurt	1 cup	8.3

Adapted from *Nutritive Value of American Foods*, Agriculture Handbook No. 456 (Washington, D.C.: U.S. Government Printing Office, 1975).

poultry, or cheese that you eat. An 8-ounce glass of milk contains 8 grams of protein. You also obtain protein from the cereals, grains, and vegetables that you eat. As you can see, your protein intake can add up very quickly to meet your needs. In fact, it is difficult *not* to meet your daily protein needs (see box).

The American Heart Association recommends no more than 6 cooked ounces of animal protein such as fish, poultry, meat, or cheese daily. This is because animal protein contains fat and because excess protein is likely to be converted into fat by the body. This is similar to the amount of protein recommended by the Self-Help Nutritional Program.

People who suffer from certain serious GI diseases—inflammatory bowel disease, Crohn's disease, pancreatic disease—may need twice as much protein, however, because absorption of nutrients from the bowel is impaired or the inflammatory stressful state eats up a lot of the body's protein (nitrogen) stores. Unless protein intake is increased, a state of "negative nitrogen balance" will result and weight loss will come from muscle as well as fat.

The Two-Week Master Program supplies more than enough protein to meet your needs, regardless of your weight or physical condition: 55 to 75 grams of protein each day, on average, depending on portion size.

Vitamin and Mineral Supplements

We need some forty vitamins and minerals to maintain health. In their proper dosages, these vitamins and minerals are necessary to promote growth, reproduction, and maintenance of cell life. The amounts needed to do this job are well supplied in a good basic diet, and most of us can obtain all the vitamins and minerals we need from food.

It's true that some nutrients in food may be lost during storage or preparation, may be improperly absorbed by the body, or may be excreted too hastily as a result of many complex factors. For this reason millions of healthy people take vitamin and mineral supplements, often in massive doses. For the most part, I believe that vitamin and mineral supplements are unnecessary. Even worse, when dosages are abused, supplements can be dangerous. Although too little of any essential nutrient can produce deficiency, too much can result in toxicity.

Fat-soluble vitamins—A, D, E, and K—are stored by the body, which means they can accumulate and become toxic if you ingest too much. High doses of vitamin A, for example, can cause bone pain and headache due to increased intracranial pressure.

Water-soluble vitamins—C and B vitamins—are rapidly absorbed and rapidly excreted. Rapid excretion in the urine means that it's hard to overdose on these vitamins, although it is possible. Megadoses of vitamin B6, for example, can cause nerve damage. When taken in large amounts, almost any nutrient becomes toxic.

Minerals are derived from metals and salts such as iron and calcium, sodium chloride and phosphorus. We need most minerals only in minute quantities and, like vitamins, excesses can do more harm than good.

• When to Take Supplements

For the majority of people with GI problems, the Two-Week Master Program supplies all the nutrients necessary and they will not require supplemental vitamins and minerals. However, there are certain exceptions. Supplemental vitamins and minerals may be good for people who have diseases such as ileitis or Crohn's disease, which are often accompanied by deficiencies. A person who has GI bleeding from ulcers may need iron supplements.

Another exception would be if you are severely cutting calories to lose weight. If your caloric intake is less than 1200 calories a day, you should take a multivitamin supplement that includes iron, as well as a calcium supplement. Certainly if you are pregnant you will probably want to take a high-potency vitamin as prescribed by your obstetrician.

Calcium supplements may be of value for women at risk for osteoporosis. Calcium has also proved beneficial for preventing colonic polyps. So if you have a family history of colonic polyps or colon cancer, you may want to take calcium supplements.

• Vitamin C and GI Disorders

Vitamin C usually does not make heartburn or ulcers worse, even though it is an acid. It doesn't seem to matter much which form of vitamin C you take. Some people think that vitamin C from rose hips is easier on the digestive system than regular ascorbic acid, but rose hips contain ascorbic acid too. If you took pure rose hips to give you a megadose of vitamin C, the pill would be the size of a golf ball. So it doesn't seem to matter to the GI tract which kind of vitamin C you ingest. Chewable ascorbic acid tablets may erode tooth enamel, so I would choose the regular tablets that you swallow whole.

Whether megadoses of vitamins, especially vitamin C, can actually promote health by preventing viral illness and cancer remains controversial. Proponents of orthomolecular medicine (which theorizes that people have inherited a biochemistry that requires very high vitamin intake, and that without supplements sickness of mind or body sets in) extol the value of 1 to 2 grams or more of vitamin C a day, but in my view convincing proof is lacking. Lack of proof hasn't stopped my wife from taking 1 gram of vitamin C a day. Having looked at the available data and had the opportunity to spend an evening with Nobel laureate Dr. Linus Pauling, she considers him too brilliant to discount. Anybody still publishing important papers on crystallography in his eighties in prestigious journals like *Nature* cannot be ignored.

One word of caution: if you decide to take large doses of vitamin C (more than 1 gram a day) you may have more frequent bowel movements or notice that your stools become looser because of its laxative effect.

*Y*our GI tract needs both macronutrients (carbohydrate, protein, and fat) and micronutrients (vitamins and minerals) to manufacture new cells. It requires essential enzymes to break down and transport food. And it requires hormones to regulate this whole process.

If the GI tract is deprived of any essential nutrients, the small intestine can shrink, which results in poor absorption, diarrhea, and increased risk of infection. Deficiencies ultimately affect every organ in the body, including the immune system. True deficiency diseases are rare because of the wide variety of foods that are available to us in the United States. (We are much more likely to suffer from overconsumption of nutrients, particularly fat.) For your body to function at peak performance over your lifetime, you need to avoid either overconsumption or underconsumption of essential nutrients.

24 *Flag Foods for Fine Tuning*

*T*he perfect GI diet would reduce the formation of stomach acid and intestinal gas, promote GI motility and proper elimination while avoiding spasms or cramps, prevent reflux of stomach acid, and reduce stimulation of the gallbladder and pancreas. Even though many people have two or more GI complaints, I've never known anyone to need all of the above features at the same time. Furthermore, people with the same symptoms may react in different ways to the same food. If the Two-Week Master Program eliminated every known gastrointestinal irritant, you might wind up with nothing to eat.

An obvious example is milk. Milk doesn't pose a problem for a person with IBS (unless that person is lactose intolerant). But milk can cause a problem for ulcer patients because it increases the production of stomach acid.

Decades of clinical research have isolated foods that tend to irritate the lining of the GI tract, cause spasm, stimulate acid secretion, or produce gas. By the time these studies circulate piecemeal through the professional medical community and trickle down to the consumer, it is impossible for the average person, or even the average doctor, to systematically apply them to a therapeutic nutritional plan.

The key to making any GI nutritional program work is to discover the specific foods that aggravate *your* particular symptoms. Flag Foods solve that problem, providing a way to personalize the Self-Help Nutritional Program.

Flag Foods are the specific foods that trigger particular GI disorders. The Flag Foods for your particular GI problem will soon become so familiar to you that they will be like bells going off any time you encounter them.

Flag Foods help you adjust the program in another important way. Different people suffering with the same GI complaint may require more severe dietary restraints than others. Flag Foods let you "tune" the Two-Week Master Program to make it more or less restrictive. If you find one of your Flag Foods listed in a recipe, you can eliminate or substitute for that ingredient when you prepare your meal. For example, those who are lactose intolerant may find that they can tolerate some milk products; others will have to eliminate milk products completely. (In the recipe section, every Flag Food carries an asterisk.)

The following lists present the Flag Foods that are specific irritants for each GI problem. To design your personal list, look under headings for your particular disorder(s).

You may find with experience that some Flag Foods on your list really don't bother you. If so, it's perfectly all right to include them in your diet. If they don't bother you, they probably aren't hurting your GI system.

Conversely, you may have a problem with certain foods that *don't* appear on your Flag Food list. Peppers, for example, may help stimulate the defense mechanism of the stomach lining, so they are not included on the Flag Food list for ulcers. If you think peppers are a problem for you, try eating them. If they bother you, add them to your Flag Foods list and avoid them in the future.

Heartburn

The Flag Foods for heartburn, sometimes called reflux esophagitis or gastroesophageal reflux disease (GERD), are listed in three categories. It is a good idea to (1) eliminate foods that relax the LES, (2) reduce foods that irritate the esophagus, and (3) reduce foods that form stomach acid and gas.

Flag Foods That Relax the LES

Fatty or greasy foods, including:
    Fried foods
    High-fat meats
    Untrimmed meats, poultry skin
    Butter, margarine, mayonnaise
    Cream, cream sauces
    Salad dressings
    Pastries, most desserts
    Whole-milk dairy products

Chocolate

Nuts

Peppermint

Caffeine-containing beverages, including:
    Soft drinks

Coffee
Cocoa
Tea

Flag Foods That Irritate the Esophagus

Alcohol

Chili powder

Black pepper

Citrus juices, including:
    Tomato juice
    Orange juice
    Grapefruit juice

Flag Foods That Produce Stomach Acid and Gas

Caffeine-containing beverages

Decaffeinated coffee

Milk, cream

Carbonated beverages

Note: Remember, if you have heartburn, avoid late-night snacks before bedtime, and try to keep the head of your bed elevated to prevent acid reflux.

Peptic Ulcer Disease

Flag Foods for peptic ulcer disease are similar to those for heartburn except that there is no need to eliminate foods that relax the LES, unless reflux is also a problem for you.

Flag Foods for Peptic Ulcer Disease

Alcohol

Chili powder

Black pepper

Citrus juices

Decaffeinated coffee

Milk, cream

Carbonated beverages

Caffeine-containing beverages

Intestinal Gas

Intestinal gas may produce flatulence, belching, or simply pain in the abdomen. All categories of food can produce gas. It's largely a matter of discovering which specific foods bother you.

Flag Foods "Hot List" for Intestinal Gas

Milk and milk products, except lactose-reduced or lactose-free

Dried beans, peas, and lentils, including soybeans

Apricots

Broccoli

Brussels sprouts

Cabbage

Cauliflower

Corn

Grapes

Prune juice

Raisins

Turnips

Nuts

Wheat germ

Wine

Food sweetened with sorbitol

Flag Foods That Cause Gas in Some People

Fruits

Bananas	Melons
Citrus fruits	Peaches
Berries	Pears
Dried fruits	Prunes
Apples, apple sauce, apple juice	

Vegetables

Asparagus	Onions
Avocado	Potatoes
Carrots	Radishes
Celery	Sauerkraut

Cucumbers	Scallions
Eggplants	Shallots
Green peppers	Tomatoes
Lettuce	Zucchini

Other

Graham crackers

Popcorn

Corn and potato chips

Soft drinks

Pastries

Wheat products

Milk Intolerance

If you suffer from milk intolerance, also called lactase deficiency, you will have to restrict your consumption of foods containing lactose. The degree of restriction varies with each person. When you begin the Two-Week Master Program, you should avoid lactose completely. Gradually, you should add small amounts of lactose to the diet while observing for symptoms of flatulence, diarrhea, and abdominal cramps.

Fermented dairy products are often well tolerated by lactase-deficient individuals and are a good source of dietary calcium, so by all means experiment with low-fat yogurt, low-fat cheese, and low-fat cultured buttermilk.

Lactaid or Lactrace, supplemental lactase enzymes, when added to milk in the recommended dose, will reduce the lactose by 70 to 100 percent.

Flag Foods "Hot List" for Milk Intolerance

Milk, skim, low-fat, or regular (except lactose-reduced or lactose-free)

Cream

Cottage cheese, ricotta cheese

Ice cream, ice milk

Flag Foods That Most People Can Use in Moderation
___
Yogurt
Aged cheese
Cultured buttermilk

Chronic Pancreatitis

Flag Foods for Chronic Pancreatitis
___
Fatty or greasy foods, including:
    Fried foods
    High-fat meats and untrimmed meats
    Butter, margarine, mayonnaise
    Cream, cream sauces
    Chocolate, pastries, most desserts
    Salad dressings
    Whole milk dairy products
High-protein foods, including:
    Nuts   Seafood
    Tofu   Peanut butter
    Meat   Poultry
    Fish   Eggs

Constipation, Diverticulosis, IBS

The following foods (except bananas) tend to cause constipation because they are usually eaten in place of unrefined carbohydrates.

Flag Foods for Constipation, Diverticulosis, IBS
___
Refined sugar
Pastries
Candy
Bananas
Baked goods made with white flour
Too much meat

People who have IBS and also have gas should also avoid Flag Foods listed for intestinal gas.

Hemorrhoids

At the first sign of a hemorrhoid attack, it might be helpful to switch to a low-fiber, low-residue diet until the acute symptoms of pain and itching subside, but you should return to the Self-Help Nutritional Program as soon as possible. The following foods are known to irritate hemorrhoids.

Flag Foods for Hemorrhoids

Any hot, spicy food
Peppers

25 Smoking, Alcohol, and Caffeine and Digestive Disorders

Smoking and GI Disorders

The premature death rate from all diseases is much higher among smokers than nonsmokers. The mechanism by which smoking affects disease and premature death is complex and in some cases not well understood, but the statistics speak out loudly, and the facts are inescapable. According to statistics first released by the American Cancer Society more than twenty-five years ago, a person who smokes two packs of cigarettes a day has a premature death rate ninety times higher than that of nonsmokers.

A recent survey by the National Institute of Health Sciences has determined that even living with people who smoke doubles a person's risk of developing cancer. The risk goes up according to how many smokers a person lives with. In fact, *smokers* living with other smokers increase their own risk of cancer, because second-hand smoke is more toxic and laden with more carcinogens than directly inhaled smoke.

Although most people know that smoking tobacco increases the risk of cancer and heart attacks, its effects on nutrition are not as well known. We know that tobacco use hinders calcium metabolism and may accelerate osteoporosis. Many smokers use cigarettes to keep from eating, and as a result may suffer nutritional deficiencies. Other substance abuse is also known to interfere with nutrition. Cocaine alters appetite, and heavy users often develop nutritional deficiencies. The same is true of heroin addicts and people who abuse other drugs.

When it comes to GI disorders, cigarette smoking is equally hazardous. Smoking makes heartburn worse by reducing the pressure of the LES and letting acid reflux more easily. Because smoking increases the urgency to defecate, it can aggravate the symptoms of IBS. Cigarette smoking also increases the likelihood of getting ulcers, especially those caused by aspirin or ibuprofen, makes ulcers harder to heal even with strong medication, and increases the likelihood that ulcers will return after healing. Finally, smoking increases the risk of cancer of the tongue, esophagus, pancreas, and bladder.

Alcohol and GI Disorders

In moderation, alcohol seems to have little harmful effect on most healthy nonpregnant adults, although some recent studies dispute this. Some studies suggest that alcohol may even have several beneficial effects: it raises HDL, the good high-density lipoproteins in cholesterol, and relieves stress by relaxing tense muscles. But if a little alcohol may be helpful, a lot can be devastating.

Alcohol contributes to 10 percent of all deaths in the United States each year, including those associated with diseases affecting the liver, heart, and other vital organs, as well as accidental death and homicide.

Women are particularly vulnerable to the ill effects of alcohol because they have lower amounts of the enzyme that breaks down alcohol in their stomachs, and therefore their bodies absorb more alcohol. This may be the reason that in women the liver, the clearinghouse for alcohol, is more readily damaged by alcohol. Pregnant women must be especially wary because alcohol easily crosses the placenta and damages the fetus. Babies born to alcoholic women are at high risk for fetal alcohol syndrome, a cluster of severe physical and mental defects that accounts for half of all birth defects. Even women who drink a modest, or perhaps any, amount of alcohol during pregnancy may increase their baby's risk of birth defects and of being born underweight.

Alcohol is one of the dietary factors most frequently associated with GI illness. Alcohol can damage the entire length of the GI tract and makes existing GI ailments worse across the board. Alcohol abuse creates a cancer risk, especially in the body parts that are exposed to the alcohol, such as the esophagus and stomach. In a study of over 8000 Japanese men living in Hawaii, those who consumed more than 16 ounces of beer daily had an increased risk of rectal cancer. Alcohol is an irritant to the stomach by damaging the stomach lining. While alcohol probably doesn't cause ulcers, it certainly can cause gastritis and can make existing ulcers worse. Because alcohol can also damage the lining of the small intestine, the absorption of nutrients may be impaired, leading to malnutrition. Even if alcoholics eat good diets they may still have nutritional deficiencies because the nutrients aren't absorbed.

Alcohol also causes various other nutritional problems. Excessive alcohol consumption interferes with metabolism and reduces appetite, leading to dangerous weight loss. Alcohol lowers blood sugar, which can lead to volatile emotions. People who drink also tend to consume quantities of caffeine, nicotine, and sugar, which can also cause wild swings in blood glucose levels.

All the alcohol you ingest must be detoxified by the liver. So if you drink, drink in quantities that the liver can handle. The liver can normally process about 1 ounce of alcohol per hour, which translates into about 4 ounces of wine, 12 ounces of beer, or 1 ounce of distilled liquor. If you drink more than that in one hour, the liver has to work harder to clear your blood of toxic alcohol. Prolonged heavy drinking can lead to chronic inflammation and eventually scarring of the liver (cirrhosis) and death. Complications from liver disease are the ninth leading cause of death in the United States.

There is really no role for alcohol in the Self-Help Nutritional Program. While many people can tolerate small amounts of alcohol on a daily basis without having significant GI symptoms, for the most part alcohol aggravates GI conditions, particularly reflux esophagitis, gastritis, peptic ulcer disease, and sometimes gallbladder disease and IBS.

Caffeine and GI Disorders

In terms of the body as a whole, caffeine appears to produce beneficial effects when used in moderation and negative effects when used in excess. When you drink a cup of coffee, the caffeine in it is absorbed immediately. The brain is stimulated and blood flow is increased to the heart. This direct effect picks you up when you feel tired, but makes you jittery when you consume too much caffeine. Caffeine raises the basal metabolic rate so your body burns calories faster. But it also triggers the release of insulin, which makes you feel hungry. Caffeine stimulates the heart muscle and can make the heart a more efficient pump. But at high doses it can cause a too-rapid heartbeat and irregular heart rhythms.

Very little good can be said about caffeine when it comes to GI problems. Caffeine relaxes the muscles of the digestive tract and blood vessels, making the kidneys increase urinary output. Thus, caffeine can dehydrate body cells. Large amounts of coffee can cause intestinal secretion and diarrhea, while the tannins in tea can cause constipation. Caffeine also promotes the secretion of acid in the stomach. One well-designed study showed that both *regular and decaffeinated* coffee can stimulate acid secretion, so ulcer patients are advised to avoid coffee in any form.

Coffee is also notorious for its ability to induce heartburn, especially if consumed on an empty stomach. Ohio State University researchers showed that this can happen even after drinking decaffeinated coffee. All coffees cause a drop in pressure in the valve at the end of the esophagus (lower esophageal sphincter, or LES). As the LES relaxes, it allows some of the acidic stomach contents to back up, producing the typical burning effects of heartburn and indigestion. The researchers related this effect not to caffeine, but to the large variety of acids, including tannic, acetic, nicotinic, formic, and citric acids, found in coffee. Tea also contains acid, in particular tannic acid, that can irritate the digestive tract. The effect of tannic acid can be countered by adding milk to tea.

Heavy coffee drinking may also cause symptoms that mimic an anxiety attack, including headache, jitteriness, upset stomach, and difficulty sleeping. Since anxiety is a trigger factor for many GI disorders, drinking coffee may set up a chain reaction: coffee leads to anxiety, anxiety leads to a reaction in the digestive system.

• Foods with Caffeine

Most obviously, caffeine is found in coffee. A 5-ounce cup of percolated coffee contains about 110 milligrams of caffeine. The same cup of coffee prepared by the drip method contains 146 milligrams of caffeine. Instant coffee, on the other hand, has about half the caffeine of regular coffee—60 milligrams in a 5-ounce cup.

On the whole, tea contains less than coffee, although some "power" teas may contain as much or even more than regular coffee. Tea brewed in bags has slightly more caffeine than loose tea, and in general, domestic brands of tea have less caffeine than the imported black teas. The longer you brew the tea, the more caffeine it contains. A cup of tea brewed with a tea bag for five minutes contains 46 milligrams of caffeine. Brewed for only one minute it contains 28 milligrams of caffeine.

Cola drinks are another source of caffeine. Although the amount of caffeine in cola drinks is much less than in coffee—ranging from 17 to 26 milligrams in 6 ounces—the serving size of soda is typically 12 ounces, which gives a caffeine dose of 34 to 53 milligrams. Cocoa and chocolate contain lesser amounts of caffeine (13 milligrams to 5 ounces).

• Alternatives to Caffeine

Decaffeinated coffee is not a useful alternative to regular coffee with regard to prevention of GI symptoms, but grain-based substitutes, such as Postum and Pero, should be all right. Some coffee substitutes are made from bran, wheat, and molasses; others are made from barley, rye, chicory, and beets. As with coffee, however, excessive consumption of grain-based products may have a laxative effect or cause flatulence.

Herbal teas may be safe substitutes for coffee, but you will need to experiment with these to see if they produce any negative effects for you. Some herbal teas can be toxic in large quantities, and all herbal teas should be used with caution.

• Breaking the Caffeine Addiction

Are you addicted to caffeine? People who consume large amounts of caffeine are likely to show their addiction by a rapidly increased heartbeat, anxiety, excess sweating, and other symptoms of stress. But you don't have to take in much caffeine to develop a caffeine habit, and you may show no outward signs of addiction. Some people who drink only one or two cups of coffee in the morning ("Just enough to get my heart started") are addicted. One quick way to tell: Skip your morning coffee, and avoid caffeine the rest of the day. If you feel well all day you are not addicted. If you start to develop severe headache and nausea by early afternoon you are addicted.

The way to break a caffeine habit without turning your system upside down is to tail off slowly. Reduce your coffee consumption by one or two cups a day until you're totally off caffeine. You may have a day or two when you feel a little groggy, but it will pass quickly, and things soon return to normal. People who give up caffeine are just as alert, and function just as well, as those who consume caffeine.

Part Six

Weight Considerations

26 *How to Adjust Calories for Your Needs*

Some of us are taller or shorter than others; some too heavy and others too thin. The Two-Week Master Program averages about 1850 calories a day—which may not be enough for some people, and may be a little too much for others. For this reason, it's important to be able to adjust the program upward or downward to suit your own needs.

Calculating Your Caloric Needs

Before making any adjustment in the diet, you should take a few minutes to discover exactly how much you should weigh and how many calories you need each day to maintain your ideal body weight.

Most people don't even come close to making an accurate assessment of how much they eat. In a study of diet histories, men underestimated their calorie intake by an average of 500 calories daily, while women missed the mark by an average of 900 calories daily. When you consider that you might need only about 1800 calories to maintain your ideal body weight, these wild guesses can become significant.

Adding Calories

If you need more calories than are provided by these meal plans, you can increase your portions and add a little more of the high-calorie foods such as margarine. If you find you are losing more weight than you wish, or if you want to gain weight, increase your portions and snack between meals on low-fat foods such as fruit, low-fat yogurt, bagels, whole-grain bread with jelly or jam, fig bars, or other low-fat cookies (see recipes). In other words, eat all of the same foods as on the Two-Week Master Program, but eat more of them.

Your Most Desirable Body Weight

Most of us know when we are at our ideal body weight. But given the changing fashion dictates of our time, as well as the social demand for thinness, it's easy to get a distorted view of just how thin we should be. People who suffer from anorexia typically have a distorted view of their bodies, seeing themselves as fat even when they are bone thin.

An easy way to find out how much you should weigh is to check a height-and-weight chart such as that provided by the Metropolitan Life Insurance Company. The problem with this table and others like it is that it's based on averages and doesn't allow for individual adjustments. You can make your own quick calculation by using the following rules of thumb.

Find Your Body Frame

Wrap your thumb and index finger around the smallest part of your wrist. If your thumb and index finger touch, you are medium build. If you cannot close your fingers around your wrist, you have a large body build. And if your fingers overlap, you have a small body build.

Find Your Body Weight

Women: 100 pounds for the first 5 feet
          5 pounds for each additional inch
          Example: 5 foot 3 inch woman
          100 pounds + (5 × 3) = 115 pounds

Men: 106 pounds for the first 5 feet
          6 pounds for each additional inch
          Example: 5 foot 11 inch man
          106 pounds + (6 × 11) = 172 pounds

Adjust for Body Build

For small body frame—deduct 10 percent from estimated weight.
For large body frame—add 10 percent to estimated weight.

Adjust for Age

If you are more than 50 years old, add 10 percent to estimated weight.

Thus, a 5 foot 3 inch woman of medium build, age 55 years old, should weigh about 115 + 11.5 (10%) = 126.5 pounds.

How Many Calories?

It's difficult to calculate how many calories you need to reach and maintain your ideal body weight, because many variables are in play. You can have your caloric needs charted by a qualified professional in a hospital, weight loss center, or exercise physiology center. The technique involves measuring oxygen consumption and carbon dioxide production. Sometimes centers use standardized formulas to calculate caloric needs. This kind of detailed calculation is usually reserved for severely malnourished or severely obese people. Most people do not need to know their caloric needs so precisely. The following formula can give you a fairly accurate ballpark figure, without investing in an expensive testing procedure. To calculate how many calories you need you first need to assess your activity level.

What Is Your Activity Level?

Sedentary—mostly sitting throughout the day: office work, studying, lab work, teaching, and no regular exercise program

Moderately active—mostly standing and walking, very little sitting in your job; or if your job is sedentary, you exercise about three times a week

Very active—daily vigorous exercise or sports

Calculate Your Calorie Needs

Sedentary—13 calories per pound

Moderately active—14 calories per pound

Very active—15 calories per pound

Thus, a sedentary woman weighing 115 pounds needs 1495 (115 × 13) calories a day to maintain her weight.

Note: If you are underweight as a result of your GI disorder and need to gain weight, be sure to read Chapter 29.

Subtracting Calories

A low-fat diet such as the Two-Week Master Program is automatically good for weight control. Most people who follow the program will lose weight or control weight easily without counting calories.

Most of the calories come from carbohydrates, which are more readily turned into energy than fat calories.

However, if the 1850-calorie level is too high for you, there are three easy ways to cut calories without losing the digestive benefits of the diet.

1   You can reduce calories most efficiently by eliminating or decreasing the added fats—margarines, mayonnaise, oil—and by using a lower-fat salad dressing. (Recipes are given in Chapter 43 for both a moderate-fat and a low-fat dressing.)

2   You can reduce the portion size of the recipes. If you do reduce portion sizes, you should make up for any possible loss of nutrients by taking a multivitamin and mineral supplement.

3   You can choose those recipes with the least fat content. Even though all GI recipes are fairly low in fat, some have almost no fat at all. Stick with those extremely low-fat recipes to give you the most nutrition for your calories. We have included the fat content in every recipe for your convenience.

All recipes in the last section of this book have their calorie content listed, and their macronutrients itemized. Every recipe and meal plan provides information about fat, protein, carbohydrate, fiber, and calorie values. This means that you can pick and choose recipes that appeal to you, meet the requirements of your GI problem, and provide the number of calories you wish to consume each day.

27 *Losing Weight*

*I*f you have GI complaints and are overweight, one of the best things you can do for yourself is shed excess pounds. Extra weight aggravates many GI problems, especially heartburn, excessive intestinal gas, belching, and gallstones. Obesity may also have a damaging effect on the liver (see Chapter 23).

Obesity is associated with many other significant health problems. If you are more than 20 percent above your ideal body weight you have a higher than normal risk of developing high blood pressure, heart disease, diabetes, high cholesterol, and several types of cancer, including colon cancer, breast and uterine cancer in women, and prostate cancer in men. Your risk is higher if you carry the extra weight around your middle than around your hips or thighs. (So you may need to exercise to get rid of a spare tire, even if you aren't obese.)

By contrast, weight control has been proved to be an important factor in lowering the risk of coronary heart disease, high blood pressure, and diabetes, and it plays an important role in any cholesterol-lowering plan. Obese individuals tend to have low HDL-cholesterol levels, the good cholesterol that helps fight heart disease. Weight loss can raise HDL cholesterol, lower the bad LDL cholesterol, and improve the cholesterol ratio.

The United Weight Control Corporation, where I am medical director, in affiliation with Thomas Jefferson University Hospital, has documented many cases in which patients have shown significant improvement in serum cholesterol, triglycerides, and blood sugar, as well as blood pressure, after losing only one-quarter of the weight they needed to lose to reach their ideal weight goal. So even modest weight loss is important for improving health.

Causes of Weight Problems

Our ability to eat almost everything and turn it into usable fuel has its down side. We have developed a taste for a bewildering variety of foods, and as a result some of us are attracted to the low end of the nutritional scale, and many of us overeat. In America one person in four is overweight.

Lifestyle influences weight problems. In a large study of families where regular activity and proper eating habits were encouraged, children had better nutritional habits and were slimmer and more active. Economics also plays a part. Large surveys show that low-income women are more likely to have a weight problem than more affluent women. Why? One might speculate that with less money to spend on quality foods and several mouths to feed, poor women purchase the least expensive and subsequently least nutritious foods. Self-image and social habits probably play a part, also. We know that people who watch a lot of television are fatter than those who don't. TV viewing burns almost no calories and encourages continuous trips to the refrigerator.

All of that being said, there's more to excess weight than eating habits and lifestyle. Several new scientific studies have shown the strong genetic basis of obesity, proving that obesity is a real disease, not a personality disorder. One large study of over 6000 adults found that overweight people did not eat more than their normal-weight peers, even when exercise levels were taken into consideration. Different people burn calories at different rates. And some people are born with more fat cells than others, which makes it easier for them to gain weight.

Fat cells are the cells that make up adipose tissue (fat). You are born with a certain number of fat cells. Overfeeding in infancy can increase weight by increasing the number of fat cells. But as an adult, the number of your fat cells is generally fixed, and weight gain occurs as the size of each fat cell increases. That's why if the fat cells are removed surgically (suction lipectomy), they tend not to come back.

Yet even with this strong new evidence pointing straight at genetics, most of us still believe that if fat people would just stop eating so much they would be thin. We assume that heavy people have less willpower than thin people. Even overweight people themselves and, more surprisingly, doctors, believe that being fat is the individual's fault and that somehow they are weak people.

People who are overweight in modern American society have a tough social scenario to live with. Thin is in, fat is out, and this social dictate appears to be securely entrenched. Overweight people, even those within ten to twenty pounds of their ideal weight, are subject to close social scrutiny. Go to any party or social gathering and listen to the immediate comments on weight gain or weight loss: "Lois, you look wonderful. Have you lost weight?" "Max, good to see you. You've put on a few pounds, haven't you?" "Jane, I feel I have to say this to you, you need to lose some weight."

We even do it to ourselves. "Sarah, how are you?" "Okay, I guess, but I've got to lose ten pounds."

Growing up with this burden of guilt can obviously be a source of great anxiety and stress. And stress caused by obesity can lead to many unpleasant symptoms such as diarrhea and heartburn and, in some cases, to actual disease such as peptic ulcers and severe psychological problems.

The causes of obesity are many and complex: genetics, faulty appetite control, poor eating habits and food choices, emotional and cultural factors. A better knowledge of nutrition and how it works, along with exercise and relaxation are the keys to healthy weight control. But many of us still turn to drastic dieting as a solution. About 34 million Americans are overweight, but at least 70 million think they should be on a diet!

Bad News Diets

At any given time, some 20 million of us actually are on some sort of weight-loss diet, and this obsession has led us into some dangerous eating habits—eating binges alternating with fasting.

People who are overweight tend to bounce from one weight-loss plan to another, doing much damage to their bodies in the process. Many very-low-calorie diets are unsafe and ultimately ineffective. Constipation and intolerance to cold can result from very-low-calorie diets. Gout, abdominal cramps, and fainting spells may result from fasting. Many of the early liquid diets provided such low-quality protein that vital body organs became starved, and in a few instances death resulted. Such diets caused depletion of important vitamins and minerals such as calcium, magnesium, sodium, and potassium, leading to disastrous shifts in electrolyte balance. The worst problem, from the dieter's point of view, is that after such struggling and deprivation they eventually regain all of the lost weight, and often more. Many studies have shown that 95 percent of those who lose weight will regain it over the next two years.

The Good News

If you are severely obese and want a formula high-quality protein diet, or a combination of food and formula, a few new programs are now available that overcome many of the problems inherent in the early very-low-calorie plans. At Jefferson we use the United Weight Control Corporation Permanence and Risk Reduction Plans for patients who are significantly obese. Since calories are not as severely restricted as in other such programs and extra fiber is added, healthy, more symptom-free weight loss is often the result. We measure body composition on a sophisticated electromagnetic scan machine at regular intervals to make sure our patients are losing fat stores rather than protein (muscle) stores. Most people can keep the weight off by entering a long-term maintenance phase after active weight loss.

Even if you try a formula diet, eventually you have to start eating regular food. Then what can you do to avoid regaining the weight you lost? First of all, take it easy—emotionally and nutritionally. Take the pressure off yourself and let it sink in that if you follow a nutritionally sound diet that benefits your digestive disorder, you will also be able to control your weight.

While the Self-Help Nutritional Program is primarily a therapeutic diet designed to prevent and treat digestive disorders, it is also an excellent weight-loss vehicle. It is high in nutrition, but lower in fat—and calories—than standard American fare. At the same time it rates high on the satisfaction scale.

Hunger is the Number One diet breaker. The high fiber content of the Self-Help Nutritional Program means that you probably won't feel hunger pangs even though you are eating less. Most people who follow the program to lose weight never feel deprived, even though they are consuming fewer calories than usual.

When you eat high-fiber foods, fluid causes the fiber to expand and occupy a greater volume in the stomach. When the stomach is distended, signals pass through nerve endings in the stomach walls, up the central nervous system to the brain, and the brain senses that you are full. Soluble fiber slows down the rate at which the stomach empties, which means that you feel fuller for a longer time. Thus, a high-fiber program provides greater satisfaction with fewer calories, a big help in reducing the stress associated with dieting. Many people on a high-fiber diet even forget they are dieting.

Because high-fiber foods are also complex carbohydrates, most people seem to lose their desire for desserts and candy. High-fiber intake lowers the level of blood insulin, which reduces your desire for food, especially sweets.

Beyond all of these weight-loss benefits, and even more important from a health standpoint, including high-fiber foods in your diet can help make weight control a permanent part of your life. Finding a way to control weight with the foods that also enhance and extend our lives is an important goal.

Fats vs. Carbohydrates

Overweight people who begin the Two-Week Master Program almost always lose weight automatically because, gram for gram, vegetables, fruits, grains, and other complex carbohydrates contain fewer calories than fats. Every gram of carbohydrate has 4 calories, while every gram of fat has more than twice that number. There are 454 grams in a pound, so a pound of carbohydrate contains 1816 calories. But a pound of fat contains 4086 calories!

By replacing fat with complex carbohydrates, you reduce calories, even though you may actually be eating *more* food. We speak of the number of calories per unit of weight as *caloric density*. Fatty food has greater caloric density than any other food. Since our program is low in fat, it has low caloric density—which means it is ideal for weight loss.

In addition, the body doesn't have to work very hard to store fat as opposed to carbohydrate. The body stores fat so efficiently that it uses only 3 calories to convert 100 calories of dietary fat into body fat. In contrast, the body must spend 23 calories to convert 100 calories of dietary carbohydrate into body fat. This means that you burn less energy after a fatty meal than after a carbohydrate-enriched meal, another factor leading to weight gain.

Overall, by concentrating on complex carbohydrates, the Two-Week Master Program is set up to give you minimum caloric density, at the same time that it forces the body to burn maximum calories to process the food it takes in.

Cutting Calories

The Two-Week Master Program provides about 1850 calories per day. If you now eat more than 3000 calories per day—and many people do—you can expect to lose a significant amount of weight on the program simply by following the recommended meal plans. If you now eat 2500 calories per day, you can expect to lose about 5½ pounds a month on the program.

If you want to lose weight but don't know how many calories you now consume every day, try this method: Begin the Two-Week Master Program, follow portion allocations carefully, and keep track of your weight twice a week. If your weight remains the same, repeat the program for two more weeks, adjusting the calorie count downward (see Chapter 6).

If you haven't lost weight after one month, consult your physician or a registered dietitian to help you design a personal weight-loss program that incorporates the principles of the program.

Diet Isn't Always Enough

Following the Two-Week Master Program is only part of a good weight-control program. Every person has a unique biochemical makeup, a preprogrammed rate at which their body burns calories. And this programming can make even the lowest-calorie diet virtually useless. A combination of your genetic makeup, the number of fat cells accumulated in your body as a child, and your current eating habits determines the weight your body would like to be. This is called "set point."

Everyone has a personal set point and it is enough to drive any dedicated dieter crazy. The more strenuously you diet, the less weight you lose as the body strives to maintain its hold on the status quo. You cut back a little more. And a little more. After several weeks of arduous calorie-cutting, you have lost a total of five or six pounds, and you can't bear the deprivation any more. You say to yourself, "If this is what it takes to lose weight, I'd rather be fat."

This set point business is part of our marvelous evolutionary advantage. When you reduce your calorie intake, your body compensates by slowing down your metabolism. The lungs use less oxygen. Cell replacement and building slow down. Vital organs reduce their demand for calories. The whole body goes into a state of semihibernation.

The set point has allowed the human species to survive periods of starvation and poor nutrition. Even now it works in our favor. For example, if you overeat on a weekend cruise, your body will start to burn calories faster because the set point speeds up your metabolism to process the unexpected excess. But if your ship goes down and you are cast adrift in a lifeboat, the set point will protect you by lowering your metabolism to burn energy slowly. Unhappily, if you cut calories on purpose to lose weight, your set point will also try to protect you against loss.

People who go off and on diets frequently are in even worse shape. Resupplied with food after a period of deprivation, the body immediately sets to work to convert as much food as possible to fat, to store up in case of yet another bout of deprivation. Yo-yo dieters tend to have a permanently slower metabolism because their set point is trying to keep things under control. They may have to restrict calories to 1000 calories a day or even less to lose weight.

Everyone wants a magic food that will effortlessly lower the set point and increase metabolism. Is it grapefruit? Is it protein? It might as well be a bird or a plane.

While the set point makes things more difficult, it is not invincible. The good news is that you can affect your body's set point and you can shake your metabolism free from its doldrums, but the magic isn't food. It's exercise.

28 Exercise to Control Weight and Improve Digestive Function

*E*xercise is the most efficient way to lower your body's set point and raise your metabolism. Exercise gives you energy, elevates your metabolism to burn fat more quickly, and lets you eat more without gaining weight. Furthermore, exercise can help people with irritable bowel syndrome and constipation because it promotes laxation and generally makes you feel better. Exercise also helps reduce stress, the great aggravator of most GI problems (see Chapter 17).

Exercise, the Mood Lifter

One great appeal of exercise, in terms of improved quality of life, is the remarkable sense of well-being it produces. Theoretically, this response is caused by the body's reaction to strong muscular activity: extra brain chemicals, called endorphins, are released to make the exertion less painful. The longer muscular effort continues, the more chemicals are released and the more euphoric you feel. These same chemicals tend to improve gastrointestinal motility.

Exercise is also a good antidote to boredom, one common reason that many of us overeat. Another interesting side benefit is that smokers who actively engage in such activities as swimming and jogging tend to quit smoking cigarettes, thereby eliminating a devastating risk factor for many life-threatening diseases, and a major culprit when it comes to digestive problems.

What Kind of Exercise?

The best exercises for helping both the heart and the digestive system are swimming, walking, and bicycling. Swimming is the least stressful of this aerobic group of exercises. Walking is better than

---

The Many Ways Exercise Helps Weight Loss

We used to believe that exercise helped weight loss simply by burning more calories. Now we know that regular exercise enhances weight loss in a host of different ways.

• Exercise burns calories. To lose a pound of fat, you must burn 3500 calories. Anything that helps burn calories is a good adjunct to dieting.

• Exercise speeds up your metabolic rate. The good effect lasts hours after you've finished exercising so that you continue to burn calories at a higher rate. If you exercise before you eat you'll benefit not only from the calories burned during exercise but from additional calories burned after the meal.

• Exercise helps control your appetite by stabilizing insulin and blood sugar.

• Exercise increases muscle mass. Muscle is the major calorie-using tissue in the body. The more muscle you have, the more food you can eat without adding body fat. Exercise maintains lean muscle tissue, tones up the body, and makes you look better and feel stronger.

• Exercise elevates your mood. Because you feel better when you exercise, it's easier to stick with your weight-loss diet.

• Exercise helps relieve stress.

• Besides helping you lose weight, exercise protects your heart by helping to lower blood pressure and cholesterol.

A special note: Exercise is clearly beneficial, but it cannot overcome the damage done by a fatty diet. You cannot get away with a steady diet of burgers, french fries, and shakes and hope to exercise off the fat and cholesterol.

---

jogging because it places minimal strain on the heels, ankles, shins, and knee joints, so the walker seldom suffers the pain of ligament damage.

A word of caution about running: recent research has confirmed what many joggers have suspected all along, that vigorous exercise, especially running, can cause heartburn even if you have not eaten recently.

Running appears to induce more reflux than exercises that involve less agitation. Dr. Don Castell, currently Director of Gastroenterology at Thomas Jefferson University, and his previous group at Wake Forest University in Winston-Salem, N.C., observed the acid levels of seven men and five women as they performed a one-hour exercise routine after a day of fasting and one hour after eating a small meal. Running consistently caused the most reflux. Weight lifting caused less reflux, and bicycling caused the least. The findings suggest that people who suffer indigestion might benefit from less jostling activities, such as bicycling.

The chest pain some people experience during exercise, which is a primary indicator of angina, may be caused by heartburn. If the chest pain is accompanied by belching or regurgitation, the problem is probably in the stomach, not the heart. However, anyone who experiences chest pain during exercise should see a doctor for evaluation and diagnosis.

How Much Exercise?

How much exercise you need to maintain health and control weight remains controversial. It appears that less rigorous workouts may be just as beneficial as strenuous activities. The continuing study of 17,000 Harvard College alumni also suggests that moderate physical exercise can increase life expectancy. In a nutshell, even moderate exercise carried out on a fairly regular basis is good for you. In terms of heart benefits, the regularity of the exercise is more important than the type of physical activity you choose. You're better off taking a brisk walk every day than playing tennis once a week. Most experts recommend a steady aerobic workout for about thirty minutes, three to five times a week.

How hard should you work out? You don't have to exercise at maximum exertion. When you must gasp for breath, the body turns up the burners on carbohydrate. That's not so good. Carbohydrates burn fast enough as it is. When you get enough air, the body uses mostly fat for fuel. That's better. So, if you must gasp to speak, you're working too hard and need to slow things down. Keep your exercise at a level that lets you speak if necessary, but not chatter on indefinitely.

Take a Walk

Walking is almost the perfect exercise, chiefly because it fits in with most people's lifestyle and can easily be carried out in a consistent manner. Walking makes the whole body function more efficiently, and there is no doubt that walking can reduce stress and improve general well-being.

CALORIES USED UP IN ONE HOUR'S WALK

Walking Speed			Your Weight in Pounds				
(miles per hour)	100	120	140	160	180	200	220
2	130	160	185	210	240	265	290
2½	155	185	220	250	280	310	345
3	180	215	250	285	325	360	395
3½	205	248	290	330	375	415	455
4	235	280	325	375	420	470	515
4½	310	370	435	495	550	620	680
5	385	460	540	615	690	770	845

Although walking won't help you lose weight fast, over time it can make a difference. The trick is to be consistent, and keep your feet moving at a brisk pace. Taking a stroll and window shopping doesn't count. Neither does meandering up and down the aisles of the supermarket, unless you're going at a dead run. A brisk one-hour walk can burn more than 300 calories an hour—the faster you walk, the more calories you burn. One-half hour of brisk walking every day can result in a 15-pound weight loss in the period of one year.

Getting Started

Regular exercise should be a part of everyone's lifestyle, yet statistics from the Centers for Disease Control show that 59 percent of Americans get less than twenty minutes of physical activity three times a week.

Many people find it hard to get started. Once they do get started, they find it difficult to continue. Part of the problem may be our perception that exercise must be performed at a specific time and in a specific place. It's true that a regular workout is ideal, but a lot of us are in the midst of playing catch-up with our daily lives. Our obligations are many, time still comes in the same twenty-four-hour allotments, and doing *anything* at precisely the same time three times a week may seem impossible. So we don't exercise at all.

If you are having trouble getting a regular program going, remember that even erratic physical activity is better than being completely sedentary. And any kind of activity is better than nothing at all. Some of us have access to gym equipment or swimming pools. Some of us enjoy sports and have the opportunity to play frequently. And some of us have none of these things. But with a little imagination it should be possible for everyone to engage in some kind of physical activity. Try to make it as regular as you can. The one thing to avoid is extreme physical exercise on an occasional basis.

Exercise will not only help you lose or control your weight, it offers very specific benefits to the GI tract. Exercise is excellent for consti-

---

Everyday Ways to Lower Your Body's Set Point

One way to begin to lower your body's set point is to sneak up on it. Think about physical activities that you enjoy and that are readily accessible to you. Dancing is good exercise, and so is table tennis. So is mopping the floor and washing the car, if you like to do it. Here are some recommendations from physical trainers of simple ways to incorporate more physical activity into daily life.

• If you work at a sedentary job, make a point of getting up every hour for a couple of minutes and walking somewhere in the office building. Climb up and down a flight of stairs, for example.

• Leave home earlier in the morning and walk to a farther bus stop than usual. On your way home, get off the bus a couple of stops before your regular stop. Instead of parking your car in the most convenient place, park it in the least convenient, the spot that makes you walk a little to reach your destination.

• Engage in at least one specific exercise session one day a week. Choose an aerobic exercise that uses your whole body. Swim or work out on a regular day, or try an exercise class at lunch hour or after work. If you get bored with the exercise you have chosen, change it. Change it every week if you like, but do some form of real exercise on your Exercise Day.

- On your Exercise Day, don't attempt too much too soon. If you choose swimming, for example, settle for doing a couple of laps the first time you go. Work up gradually until you reach the time and distance where you feel most comfortable. If you get one regular Exercise Day started and it feels good, increase it to two and then three days when you're ready.

- Run through a series of easy stretching exercises or calisthenics when you get out of bed in the morning.

- Take a brisk walk every day, no matter how brief.

- Buy a stationary exercise bike or a treadmill for your use at home. (Make sure you remember to get on it.) If you use an exercise bike, you may have to take short frequent breaks when you first begin. But if you stick with it you can extend your riding time until eventually you will be cycling more than you are resting.

- Try to find a sport you like to play. If you are competitive by nature (Type A's take heed), make sure you take it easy on your opponents until you get into good condition. Then go for it.

- After every exercise session, no matter what it is, take a little time to completely relax physically.

pation because it improves bowel function. (But marathon runners may get diarrhea because vigorous exercise can improve bowel function *too* much.) Because it helps relieve stress, exercise may decrease the incidence of ulcers and the symptoms of IBS.

There is a triad of good health prescriptives that goes like this: weight control, exercise, and stress reduction. They are interrelated. Exercise and weight maintenance are closely tied together. Exercise and stress relief are also closely linked. And all three components can have considerable impact on your health, particularly your risk for heart disease and GI problems. Of the three, stress is the most mysterious, and the most critically involved with digestive problems.

A Word of Caution

If you are over the age of thirty-five or if you have a family history of heart disease, you should consult your physician before starting an exercise program. Also, if you are in very poor condition, if you are a heavy smoker, seriously overweight, or under treatment for a medical condition, check with your doctor before embarking on an exercise regimen. You may first need to undertake supervised exercise with a trainer to work yourself into better condition. If you haven't done any physical exercise in a while, be certain to start off slowly and gradually increase your tolerance.

Don't ever go from a resting state to hard exercise. Warm-up exercises are essential to get muscles working. Similarly, after exercise, cool-down exercises will keep muscles relaxed and warm until they are fully rested.

If you feel sick or dizzy, feel a tightness in your chest, get a severe headache, or see spots, stop exercising at once and check with your doctor as soon as possible. You may have an underlying problem that needs treatment. Never push yourself beyond what feels reasonable. Exercise is never better if it hurts. After an exercise session you should feel invigorated, not devastated.

29 *If You Need to Gain Weight*

Believe it or not, some people have a problem maintaining adequate weight. Many people are thin for genetic reasons—that's just the way they are and it is normal for them. Thinness can also be caused by poor eating habits. Many underweight people eat virtually nothing throughout the day and only a small meal at night. Erratic eating habits are another common cause. Sometimes people become underweight because, under temporary stress or illness, they just stop eating.

These kind of weight-loss problems are usually fairly easy to correct. But sometimes weight loss can be a symptom that requires special attention because it can signify a serious underlying disease state.

Unexplained Weight Loss

Many digestive problems can prevent nutrients from being absorbed and properly used. Any serious disease—cancer, severe lung, heart, or kidney disorder—can cause loss of appetite and weight loss. In fact, weight loss can be caused by virtually any disease of any body system. Severe depression, for example, may lead to weight loss. (A little stress may make us eat more, but a lot of stress often makes us lose our appetite.) Anorexia nervosa, a kind of self-induced starvation undertaken by some women who perceive themselves as fat no matter how thin they become, also leads to dangerously low weight levels.

Just as obesity can create digestive problems, too little weight is also a feature of some GI problems. Because the digestive tract is responsible for the intake, digestion, and processing of food, it is not surprising that when things go wrong with the tract itself, weight loss is sometimes a by-product.

• Painful Swallowing

In many cases, weight loss is caused by poor intake of food. For example, heartburn may be so severe that swallowing becomes painful, or certain foods burn on the way down, so people stop eating. The Self-Help Nutritional Program can help relieve acid reflux and so alleviate painful swallowing.

If scar tissue builds up inside the esophagus and causes narrowing it may be difficult to swallow solid foods. Liquids may go down fairly well, but any food particle larger than the esophageal opening will stick. Weight loss may be a result.

Difficult swallowing can also occur if the esophagus doesn't contract properly. The esophagus may look perfectly normal, but instead of squeezing ingested foods along in an orderly fashion, it may contract erratically, causing food to stick along the route. With this kind of problem, known as a motility disorder, even liquids may cause difficulties. Drug therapy is often needed to control the spasm. The Self-Help Nutritional Program can also help by preventing the acid reflux that triggers the spasm.

Difficulty swallowing can also be caused by tumors of the esophagus, so it is important to see your doctor for any swallowing problems.

• Early Satiety

Weight loss can also be caused by stomach disorders. In this case a hungry person feels full after eating only a small amount. The stomach, which acts as a reservoir, is designed to expand to accommodate food. Stomach tumors make it difficult for the stomach to expand; therefore an early feeling of fullness is a common symptom. Some people always eat small meals, but if you notice a change in your eating pattern, it's important to pay attention. People who have long-standing diabetes may also develop early satiety and weight loss due to defective emptying of the stomach.

Early satiety and difficult swallowing are two important symptoms that require prompt evaluation by a physician because they may be caused by serious underlying disease.

• A Damaged Small Intestine

Any damage to the small intestine can affect food absorption and lead to weight loss. Crohn's disease (ileitis) and gluten-sensitive enteropathy (sprue), a wheat allergy, are two examples. Diseases of the small intestine can be quite serious. In mild disease, the Self-Help Nutritional Program may be helpful. But for most patients, treatment involves a highly individualized dietary and medical regimen designed by a physician working closely with a nutritionist. (In severe Crohn's disease, for example, the patient may have to be fed intravenously at first, then with improvement eventually progress to a low-residue, low-lactose, low-fat diet.)

Diseases of the large intestine generally do not cause weight loss because by the time food reaches the colon most of the nutrients have been absorbed. Only if the condition is severe enough to cause general sickness throughout the body, as in colon cancer or severe colitis, is weight loss likely to result.

How to Gain Weight

When otherwise healthy people are underweight the problem can usually be corrected by stabilizing eating patterns so that they eat three meals a day, and increasing calorie intake. This does not mean adding empty calories found in desserts and junk foods. It means concentrating on foods that are high in vitamins, minerals, *and* calories. Examples are whole grains, nuts, seeds, and dried fruits. Those following the Self-Help Nutritional Program can increase their portions and concentrate on the recipes that are somewhat higher in calories. For example, sweet potatoes have twice as many calories as white potatoes and supply even more vitamin A and minerals. Avocados are also high in calories and nutrients.

Dietary Supplements

Some people with digestive disorders associated with weight loss may need more than the Self-Help Nutritional Program. A wide variety of dietary supplements, with varying amounts of protein, fat, and lactose, are on the market, each designed to help overcome a specific nutritional and digestive problem. A supplement may be high in fiber or low in fiber. It may be high in fat or low in fat. Supplements are selected to match the individual's medical and nutritional needs. For example, certain conditions require extra protein. Some require a low-fiber, low-residue supplement. Some need extra fat, and others must be wary of cholesterol.

If you are underweight because of any medical problem and require supplements to maintain body weight, it is essential that you contact your physician or a registered dietitian—or both—to make sure you choose the correct supplement for your condition.

Part Seven

═══════════════════════════════════

Your Gastrointestinal Maintenance Plan

30 *Keeping Track of Your Progress*

*T*he goal of the Self-Help Nutritional Program is to reduce the frequency and severity of GI symptoms. The more frequent and severe the symptoms before starting the diet, the easier it will be to measure the results. Relief from milder symptoms usually cannot be measured in such a dramatic manner. However, measuring your success with the program is a good way to motivate yourself and maintain your success.

The best way to assess your progress is to keep a diary of your symptoms before and after starting the Two-Week Master Program. This doesn't mean that you will have to make diary entries forever. Keep the diary for several days before starting the program to get an average "baseline." After starting the program, continue to maintain the diary for two full weeks. This way you can easily determine how much progress you are making.

When you have completed the first two weeks, continue to incorporate the principles of the Master Program into your normal eating routine, and continue to keep track of your progress in your diary. At first you may feel compulsive about making entries, tracking even minor symptoms. Eventually, you will probably slow down and record only those symptoms that seem significant to you.

The diary will help you maintain your motivation after your symptoms have decreased. When you are feeling well and are free of pain and discomfort, it's easy to believe that it was always thus. Looking at your diary occasionally will help you remember what it was like before you started the Self-Help Nutritional Program.

Charting Your Progress

To begin, note the times of day you eat. Then record the symptoms as they occur.

Use any code that's easy for you. We use simple initials to denote:

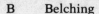

B   Belching
C   Constipation
Cr   Cramps
D   Diarrhea
F   Flatulence
H   Heartburn
P   Pain

DAY_____

12_____6_____12_____6_____12
Midnight   a.m.   Noon   p.m.   Midnight

Here's an example of how to use the daily chart. Bill suffered from gastroesophageal reflux disease (GERD). He would wake up in the middle of the night coughing and have a sour taste in his mouth. His voice was hoarse. He would get heartburn when he lay down and when bending over. He also suffered from frequent belching.

Before starting the Two-Week Master Program, Bill's daily chart looked like this:

DAY_September 30, 1989_____

Coughing   H   B B   H   H
         ↓   ↓   ↓ ↓   ↓   ↓
12   ↓   ↓   6   ↓ ↓   12   ↓   6   ↓   12
Midnight   a.m.   Noon   p.m.   Midnight

After one week on the program, antacids, and elevation of his bed, his chart looked like this:

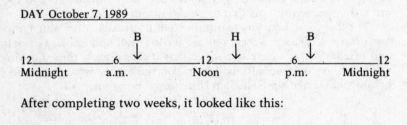

DAY_October 7, 1989_____

                    B   H   B
                    ↓   ↓   ↓
12_____6___↓_____12___↓_____6__↓_____12
Midnight   a.m.   Noon   p.m.   Midnight

After completing two weeks, it looked like this:

DAY_October 14, 1989_____

                                    B
                                    ↓
12_____6_____12___↓_____6_____12
Midnight   a.m.   Noon   p.m.   Midnight

Working with Your Doctor

The proper diagnosis and treatment of your digestive problem, as well as preventive maintenance, depends on a close, open, and effective working relationship between you and your doctor. This is true whether your doctor is a general practitioner, family physician, or internist, or a specialist in digestive diseases. You and your doctor are partners in the care of your GI disorder.

• Your Responsibilities as Patient

See Your Doctor When Symptoms Develop. It always amazes me how some people will take their pet to the veterinarian at the drop of a hat, or their child to a pediatrician at the first sniffle, but ignore potentially serious symptoms of disease in themselves. Part of this is a normal denial that we are sick, or an irrational feeling of being immortal. Some people don't like to spend money on themselves, and put their needs low on the priority list. In the case of some men, it's a case of "macho men don't get sick." This is particularly unfortunate when it comes to GI disorders because men tend to have more serious organic causes of GI disease than women do. So when symptoms occur, see your doctor now rather than later.

Be As Open As Possible with Your Doctor. Your description of your symptoms is 80 percent of the diagnosis. When it comes to GI disorders, your doctor usually cannot find out what's wrong with you just by tapping on your chest or pushing on your stomach. You need to describe your problem in detail. Don't withhold information because you think it's insignificant. Or embarrassing. No matter how embarrassing the symptoms, you must tell your doctor in order to get a diagnosis based on all the facts.

Question Your Doctor. It's important for you to understand the nature of your problem, why you need certain tests, and what they are like, including potential risks. Ask your doctor about the safety and effectiveness of any medication prescribed and what side effects to look out for.

Ask your doctor if you should alter your diet, and whether a high-fiber, low-fat diet like the Self-Help Nutritional Program would be helpful for your particular condition.

Remember, an informed patient is a good patient, someone who is more likely to experience a positive result. When it comes to GI disorders that require lifetime maintenance to avoid symptoms, your full cooperation and understanding are crucial.

Follow Your Doctor's Recommendations. It's important for you to be as compliant as possible with your doctor's recommendations. It's fairly common for patients to come to our hospital after not improving on treatment instituted elsewhere. Often the diagnosis was correct, the treatment plan was correct, but somewhere along the way a breakdown in communications occurred, and the patients weren't doing what they were supposed to do. When it comes to GI disorders, a patient has to take most of the responsibility for the treatment program. Some people may subconsciously want to maintain their sick role because of the secondary gains that are associated with being sick (more attention, relief from household chores, etc.). While these secondary gains may seem attractive in the short term, ultimately maintaining a healthy mind and body will make you a more happy and successful person.

• Responsibilities of Your Doctor

See You As Soon As Possible When You Have Symptoms. If you have serious symptoms like profuse rectal bleeding, vomiting of blood, severe abdominal pain, jaundice, or fever and chills, you should call your doctor immediately. If the doctor's secretary gives you an appointment two weeks down the road, that is inappropriate. Ask to speak to the doctor; if you cannot be seen right away, you may be directed to an emergency room.

On the other hand, if your complaint is belching, flatulence, or lifelong constipation that hasn't recently changed, waiting a few weeks for an appointment is probably medically safe.

Be Nonjudgmental. You should feel comfortable telling your doctor all of your problems. Doctors need to know about intravenous drug abuse, homosexuality, and other behavior associated with high risk for diseases such as hepatitis, chronic diarrhea, and AIDS.

Allow Enough Time. If the doctor doesn't allow enough time for an open exchange, much important information may be lost. Furthermore, if your doctor tries to direct the conversation, you may never get to some points you want to make. Doctors tend to do this at times to avoid listening to the details of every morsel of food a patient has eaten in the last week or to an entire treatise devoted to bowel function. However, important details are often embedded in these long exhortations. If you tend to be long-winded, unfocused, or just have difficulty talking to your doctor—or if your doctor tends to rush you —make a list of the things you think are important prior to your visit. That way you won't forget anything important, and your doctor won't be able to ignore the points you have written down.

The goal is to develop a smooth working relationship with your doctor, rather than an adversarial one.

Inform You About Tests. Your doctor should inform you in detail about the diagnostic tests recommended, their necessity, discomfort, risk, cost, and likelihood of making a difference in the outcome of the problem.

Design a Therapeutic Plan. An important part of your doctor's job is to formulate a therapeutic plan that is realistic for you. Asking a patient with hemorrhoids to take eight sitz baths a day is impractical if that person has a full-time job.

The treatment plan should include nutritional management in addition to drug therapy.

Keep Track of Your Progress. Your doctor should follow up on your treatment to make sure you are improving and that the working diagnosis was correct.

As you can see, if you have a GI disorder, working with your doctor is more than just making an appointment, taking some pills, and going back to your normal life. Successful diagnosis and management of a GI problem so that impairment is minimized and healthy function maximized depends on an open and trusting doctor-patient relationship.

31   *Your Everyday Cooking*

*T*he following tips about shopping and food preparation will help you incorporate the principles of the Two-Week Master Program into your everyday cooking. With a little experience you will be able to adapt your favorite recipes, and even invent new ones.

Increase Fiber

Take a trip to your local health food or bulk food store and stock up on whole grains. Brown rice, whole wheat pasta, bulgur wheat, buckwheat, whole wheat couscous, wheat berries, whole wheat flour, whole grain cereals, and whole oat products are some choices you might make. As the demand has increased, many supermarkets have also begun to carry more whole grain products.

Gradually begin to use more of these products in your cooking. Many of the recipes in the Two-Week Master Program include more whole grains than you may be accustomed to, and it's wise to make a gradual transition. If you are unaccustomed to cooking with whole grains, you may need to experiment a little with recipes to see how various grains react to the cooking process.

Also begin to increase your intake of fruits and vegetables. Begin to center meals around grains and vegetables, deemphasizing the animal protein portion of the meal. Get in the habit of using fruit as a dessert. And use the leftovers of the grain and vegetable portion of your dinner to make lunch the next day. The meal plans are designed to make use of leftovers as brown-bag meals.

Reduce Fats

Fats are typically added to diets in the form of butter, margarine, oil, mayonnaise, cream, nondairy cream, and salad dressing. Whole-milk dairy products, animal protein foods, nuts, seeds, and bakery goods are also sources of excess fat. It's easy to replace most of these items with healthier, low-fat alternatives.

Fats in Baking and Cooking. It's difficult to bake without using any fat, but much of the fat used in baked goods can be replaced with fruit, pureed fruit, or fruit juice. Many of the recipes in this book demonstrate this concept.

Fats also can be reduced by increasing the use of cooking liquids. For example, you can "sauté" using vermouth, wine, defatted broth, tomato juice, low-sodium soy sauce, fruit juice, vegetable oil sprays, or any other nonfat liquid. Jellies, jams, and fruit butters can be used in place of margarine or butter on bread. Try low-fat yogurt instead of mayonnaise, or use half yogurt and half low-fat mayonnaise. Try the lower fat salad dressing recipes included here, or purchase a bottled low-fat dressing. Try mock sour cream (see Chapter 43) instead of sour cream on your baked potato.

Soon you may be able to use "fake fats"—cooking ingredients that look and taste like fat but are either a special nonabsorbable protein (Simplesse, made by the Nutrasweet Company) or complex sugar with nonabsorbable fatty acids (Olestra, made by Procter and Gamble).

Butter and Oil. Since you will be using fat in smaller amounts, you might freeze your butter or margarine to make them last longer. Likewise, refrigerate your vegetable oils to prevent them from becoming rancid. Olive oil will thicken and may turn cloudy when refrigerated, but will return to its normal state at room temperature with no harm done.

Dairy Products. All the dairy products you use in your daily cooking—including cottage cheese, yogurt, and milk—should be low-fat. Skim or 1% low-fat is recommended; 2% low-fat and whole milk are less acceptable. Cheeses should be used only in moderation. Even cheeses partially made with skim milk are not actually low in fat.

Frozen desserts vary in their fat content and can be very misleading. Ice cream is usually high in fat; ice milk is lower, but is not low in fat. Sherbet, sorbet, and fruit ices are lower in fat. Sherbet, which is made with milk, is not lactose-free, but sorbets and fruit ices are. Frozen yogurt may be low in fat, but check the label. Likewise, tofu frozen desserts may be low in fat, but many have vegetable oils added. Read the label to be sure. Tofu-based products are lactose-free.

Animal Fats.   Meat, poultry, fish, seafood, pork, and eggs are all animal proteins. Limit your consumption of animal protein to 6 to 8 ounces a day, in keeping with the overall concept of reducing animal protein and increasing complex carbohydrates.

You can further reduce the fat content of animal protein by following a few simple rules: skin poultry before cooking, cut off visible fat from meat, and use cooking methods that help remove fat—broiling, roasting, poaching, baking, steaming, or braising.

Nuts and Seeds.   Nuts and seeds are high-fat foods that should be used only as a garnish. Nuts and seeds are also gas producing, so many people will want to avoid them completely.

Reduce Lactose

All milk and milk products contain lactose. If you are lactose intolerant, or don't know if you are, use the dairy products recommended in Chapter 20.

Even people who are lactose intolerant can usually tolerate small amounts of lactose in prepared foods. Usually these small amounts should come from cheese because fermented dairy products are often better tolerated. Yogurt is usually well tolerated by lactose-intolerant people as long as it has an active culture. Look for nonfat or low-fat yogurt with active cultures.

Substitute Herbs for Spices

Herbs can be used in place of spices in your everyday cooking. Add a small amount, taste, and add more to please your own taste. Herbs are fragile, so are usually added near the end of the cooking time.

Store herbs in a cool, dark cabinet. (Forget about the shelf above the stove where heat and light quickly destroy their flavor.) If possible purchase herbs in a shop with a high product turnover so packages haven't been sitting for months on the shelf. Herbs available in bulk almost always taste better than prepackaged varieties. They will usually be fresher and less expensive. Bulk herbs are usually sold in ½- to 1-ounce portions, and you can easily store them in your own containers. Herbs can make a tremendous difference in flavor when you use few spices and less fat, so it's important to buy top quality. Seasonal fresh herbs are especially good. Better yet, start your own herb garden.

Reduce Legumes

Legumes such as dried beans and lentils are very healthy and good for you, but they are gas forming. However, if your GI problem is not aggravated by gas, eat legumes as often as you want. Many people find that if they add small quantities of legumes to their diet several times a week their digestive systems adjust and produce less gas.

Lentils and split peas are the most easily tolerated. It also helps prevent gas if you discard the soaking liquid or the liquid legumes are canned in before using.

To Cook or Eat Raw

In general, the more you cook something the more vitamins and minerals are lost, especially the B vitamins and vitamin C. So for the most part, the less you cook vegetables the better. That being said, there are some exceptions.

Some plant foods must be cooked in order to burst the cell wall and derive nutrients from the food. Potatoes are an example. Raw potatoes provide little more than fluid and fiber. Cooked potatoes provide fluid, fiber, complex carbohydrates, vitamins, minerals, and some protein.

Carrots and beans are another example of high-fiber foods that do better if they are cooked longer. When they are cooked adequately these vegetables are more easily digested, and therefore their nutrients are better absorbed. This more efficient use of the food offsets some loss of nutrients in the cooking process.

*T*he recipes in Part Eight will give you the experience you need to begin to modify all of your cooking and eating habits.

32 *Dining Out*

When it comes to dining, no man or woman is an island. Eating is our most social activity, usually performed in the company of anywhere from one to hundreds. Every occasion, great or small, is marked by a ritual sharing of food and drink. It could be a raise or a new job, birth, engagement, wedding, shower, confirmation, bat or bar-mitzvah, graduation, new apartment or house, anniversary, retirement, or even death; it could be a picnic, potluck dinner, power breakfast, business lunch, romantic supper at an out-of-the way restaurant, or a catered affair. You get the idea. No event passes without celebration by breaking bread together. It has always been so. Our prehistoric ancestors gathered together around fires in front of caves to share the rewards of the hunt and celebrate the fact that yet another day had passed safely.

Celebrating life by sharing food is impossible to avoid for everyone but the most determined hermit. And this essential part of being human is one of our healthiest, most positive traits. But for people with GI problems, these events have often been uncomfortable or downright torture.

Let's assume you have carefully worked out your own diet, including the specific Flag Foods that you know will aggravate your GI problem. Deviating from that diet may not be dangerous, but taking a night off or splurging at lunch will often cause a reaction. It isn't so difficult to maintain your diet even at a party or a restaurant. It just takes some forethought.

Dinner Parties

We are all more nutrition and weight conscious these days than ever before in history. As a result, any get-together of two or more people is bound to include someone who has restrictions on his or her diet. It may be on a physician's advice or self-imposed, but there are many millions of people who avoid certain foods that they believe are harmful.

Today's party givers want their guests to enjoy themselves, and one thing that means is being flexible about menus. With so many health-conscious people, even cocktail parties that used to have only potato chips, dip, and peanuts for sustenance, now are likely to feature baskets of fresh vegetables, whole grain breads, and flavored seltzer as well as martinis.

One thing for you to bear in mind if you suffer from a GI disorder: managing diet at a dinner party or a restaurant is not just a whim or self-indulgence or a way to draw attention to yourself. It's as important for you to control your diet as it is for someone who is trying to manage diabetes or heart disease. You are entitled to be served foods that you can eat without becoming ill. At the same time, you don't want your host to have to do handstands to accommodate you.

So when the invitation to a dinner party arrives, it's a good idea to call your hosts and ask them for a general idea of what will be served. You can do this whether you know your hosts well or not at all. This is not so you can dictate the menu, but so you can prepare yourself in advance. By all means, explain why you're asking: you have to follow a somewhat restricted diet for medical reasons.

Obviously, if you're invited for a fish fry or a barbecue you aren't going to ask them to change the menu for your sake. But if your hosts are still preparing the menu, they are likely to ask you what restrictions you have and you can tell them in advance what your Flag Foods are.

What you don't want to do is arrive at a dinner party and spring your special dietary needs on an unsuspecting host at the last minute. I'll never forget one guest arriving at a dinner party that featured a main course of lamb navarin and announcing that he was a vegetarian. His host rushed frantically into the kitchen and prepared a vegetable and pasta dish while trying to serve dinner to eight other people.

So, if you are going to make your needs known, make them known with plenty of time to spare. Most people will be pleased to know in advance what foods their guests have to avoid.

If the menu is already set, you will know beforehand what you can eat plenty of and what you will have to stay away from. Even at the barbecue there are likely to be baked potatoes and vegetables. If it looks as if your selection is going to be severely restricted, you might want to have a snack before the party so you won't be tempted to wolf down food that will bring on an adverse reaction.

This may seem odd to you. But after all, if Scarlett O'Hara ate before the barbecue, why shouldn't you? In fact we go to dinner parties for a lot of reasons other than the food. Parties are enjoyable social occasions whether you eat much or not. Unless you're willing to eat something that's likely to trigger a GI reaction, fill yourself up beforehand on foods that you know are in line with your diet.

Fortunately, today's parties are often semibusiness engagements that are designed to satisfy a wide variety of special needs. Having a wide choice of such things as vegetables and interesting breads as well as a main course is one way for a host to make sure even the most finicky guests have something to eat.

One Los Angeles caterer always makes sure that there is plenty of extra-virgin olive oil, vegetables, fish, and plain fruit, which can satisfy most palates and stomachs. A New York caterer says the best hosts try not to serve pork, lamb, duck, or fried foods. They serve starches such as pasta, potatoes, and bread along with salad and vegetables and fruit for dessert.

Platter service, which allows guests to discreetly select what they're going to eat, and buffets, which offer variety, are popular today across the country. So chances are if you are invited to a party you will be able to manage pretty well. Restaurant dining, however, may require some skill on your part.

Restaurants

Dining in a restaurant used to be a special occasion, often to mark an important event in one's life. Today eating out is more likely to be an everyday event in many people's lives. What with lunches at restaurants near your workplace and more elaborate business lunches, Americans eat about one meal in three in restaurants.

Although many meals are eaten in fast-food restaurants where the selection is generally pretty limited and the accent is more on "fast" than "food," there is still a good chance that in most restaurants, even with GI problems, you can get a healthful, tasty meal without suffering afterward.

The same kind of forethought is necessary with restaurant meals as with partygoing. First of all, what sort of restaurant are you going to? Fast-food restaurants will not have a variety of foods for people on restrictive diets. Many items on the fast-food menu are high in saturated fats, from hamburgers with mayonnaise to french fries cooked in beef fat and shakes thickened with coconut oil. Even the fish and chicken dishes are often fried.

Most ethnic restaurants, on the other hand, have a much fresher and healthier selection of dishes for people with GI problems. This comes as a big surprise for many people who thought they would never be able to eat flavorful, tasty food again. But contrary to what you might believe, ethnic restaurants are definitely on your "go" list.

Chinese, Japanese, Mexican, Middle Eastern, and Italian restaurants all have many freshly prepared dishes that are high in fiber and low in saturated fat. Some people, depending on their Flag Foods, will have to avoid the spicier items, but even Mexican restaurants serve fish and rice dishes that are low in spice. All so-called peasant cuisines are based on combinations of inexpensive grains and vegetables that make complete dishes, high in complex carbohydrates and low in saturated fat.

It is best for anyone who has dietary restrictions to plan ahead. Restaurants are in business to give service along with good food. Call the restaurant you are planning to dine in and check out the menu over the phone. In a good restaurant you can talk to the manager or head waiter about your dietary restrictions. They will be happy to help you plan a meal that will be both satisfying to your palate and easy on your GI system.

Many people these days dine out on the spur of the moment, in a casual neighborhood restaurant or other restaurant where you really can't call ahead and do any special ordering. In this case make it a habit to ask for low-fat dairy products and foods prepared without fats or salt. Ask for the sauces and salad dressings to be served on the side so you can control the amounts you use.

More important than these special requests is making a good selection to begin with. It helps to know as much as possible about the preparation of food and the language commonly used to describe dishes on restaurant menus. If you cook, you're ahead of the game, because you understand what goes into the preparation of most dishes. If you don't cook and are unfamiliar with cooking terms and food preparation, here's a quick course in menu terminology.

Menu Terminology to Watch Out For

French

aioli: garlic mayonnaise
beurre: butter
béarnaise: sauce of egg yolks and butter with herbs and shallots
béchamel: cream sauce (flour, milk, butter)
hollandaise: sauce of egg yolks and butter with lemon

Italian

pancetta: Italian bacon
burro: butter
olio: oil
parmigiano: Parmesan cheese
formaggio: cheese
frittata: omelet

Indian

samosa: small pastry
paratha: fried bread
poori: fried bread
ghee: clarified butter

Japanese

tempura: batter-coated deep-fried fish, shrimp, or vegetables

Good Menu Choices

Salads, dressings on the side

Melon, berries, other fresh fruits

Seafood cocktails (sauce on side)

Oysters or clams on half-shell

Broth or tomato based soups with noodles or vegetables

Gazpacho (will usually have onions and/or garlic)

Minestrone (usually has beans)

Clam chowder (Manhattan style)

Tomato juice (except for people with heartburn)

Fish, all varieties, broiled, poached, or steamed

Poultry (skin it before you eat it)

Red meat, lean cuts, broiled

Vegetables, all kinds (avoid broccoli, corn, cauliflower, cabbage, fried potatoes)

Pastas, brown rice, and whole grains, all kinds, plain or with tomato sauces, wine sauces, fish and seafood sauces, vegetables

Breadsticks, hard rolls, French and Italian bread, pita bread, whole wheat toasts, and whole grain breads

Angel food cake

Gelatin

Sorbet

Low-fat dairy products (lactose intolerant individuals should bring lactase enzyme tablets with them when dining out)

Part Eight

Gastrointestinal-Healthy Recipes

33 *Appetizers and Soups*

Acorn Squash Soup

Basic Chicken Stock

Crab and Potato Chowder

Winter Vegetable Soup

Salmon Mousse

Tomato Basil Soup

Turkey Meatball Soup

Acorn Squash Soup
SERVES 4

This is a very elegant yet healthy "cream" soup. It's a great way to serve squash to those of us who are not squash lovers.

½ tablespoon butter or margarine
1 small onion, chopped
*2 garlic cloves, chopped
½ teaspoon ground coriander
¼ teaspoon ground cumin
*⅛ teaspoon ground black pepper
2 medium-sized acorn squash (about 1½ pounds total), peeled and coarsely chopped

1½ cups chicken stock, preferably homemade (see page 208)
1½ cups water
1 teaspoon sugar
1 teaspoon salt (omit if you used canned chicken broth)
**½ cup evaporated skimmed milk
*grated nutmeg

* Garlic, black pepper, and nutmeg must be avoided by many of you. The soup is quite acceptable even when they are omitted.
** If you are lactose intolerant, you may make low-lactose evaporated skimmed milk. Use two times your usual amount of lactase enzyme drops. The soup is also quite good without the milk, but the milk does add an extra dimension.

1   Melt butter in medium saucepan over medium high heat. Add onion, garlic, and spices and sauté for about 2 minutes. Add squash and stir to coat, about 1 minute. Add stock, water, sugar, and salt. Bring to a boil, turn heat to low, cover, and let simmer until squash is tender, about 10 to 15 minutes.

2   Allow squash to cool slightly and then puree in a blender or food processor.

3   Stir in evaporated skimmed milk and reheat, but do not allow to boil. Garnish with grated nutmeg and serve.

*Nutritional information per serving**

171 calories	9% of calories from fat
77% of calories from carbohydrate	2 grams of fat
14% of calories from protein	5 grams of fiber

Basic Chicken Stock

YIELD: 5 TO 6 QUARTS

Defatted stock is a wonderful basis for low-fat cooking. It is rich and flavorful but virtually fat-free. Canned broth can be used as a substitute as long as it is first defatted (refrigerate the can overnight), but the results will not be as good. Homemade stock takes a long time to make, but it is not labor-intensive time, so you can make it while you are at home doing other things. Bones and chicken scraps can be obtained inexpensively from your butcher, or if you bone your own chicken, simply save the bones, skins, and scraps in a plastic bag in your freezer. You do not need to follow this recipe exactly; use vegetables and spices that are available to you, put them in a large stock pot with the chicken, and simply cover with cold water.

about 2½ pounds chicken bones, skins, scraps	3 celery stalks and leaves, washed
	3 bay leaves
2 medium carrots, washed, unpeeled, cut into quarters	several parsley sprigs
	several dill sprigs
2 medium onions, washed, unpeeled, cut in quarters	1 teaspoon dried thyme
	1 teaspoon dried tarragon
1 leek, green and white parts, well scrubbed	20 peppercorns (if desired)
	3 garlic cloves, peeled (if desired)

1   Put all of the above into a large stock pot. Cover with cold water (probably about 6 to 7 quarts). Cover pot.

2   Turn heat to medium high. Bring to a bare simmer, turn heat to medium low.

* Throughout this section, assume that one serving is based on the number served.

3 Simmer at this temperature for 3 to 6 hours. Skim if necessary.

4 Strain. Cool in refrigerator for several hours and remove hardened fat.

5 Freeze in various size containers, including ice cube trays. Remove from the ice cube trays when frozen and store in a plastic bag in your freezer. Use these cubes for fat-free "sautéing."

Nutritional information per serving (1 cup)

26 calories

16% of calories from carbohydrate

84% of calories from protein

0% of calories from fat

0 grams of fat

0 grams of fiber

This is an approximate analysis and is based upon a *defatted* chicken stock (see step 4).

Crab and Potato Chowder

SERVES 6

1 tablespoon butter or margarine

2 leeks, well washed and finely chopped

2 cups dry vermouth

1 cup water

1½ pounds red potatoes, scrubbed, skin on, cut into bite-sized pieces

1 teaspoon salt

½ teaspoon dried thyme

*1 can (12 or 13 ounces) evaporated skimmed milk

**1 cup skim milk

1 pound crabmeat

2–3 tablespoons chopped parsley

1 Melt butter over medium high heat in 3-quart saucepan. Add leeks, turn heat to low, cover, and allow to cook slowly for 3 to 4 minutes or until softened.

2 Add vermouth, water, potatoes, salt, and thyme. Bring to a boil. Turn heat to low, cover, and cook until potatoes are fork tender, about 20 minutes.

3 Add milk and crabmeat. Heat through but do not boil. Sprinkle with chopped parsley and serve.

Nutritional information per serving

310 calories

59% of calories from carbohydrate

29% of calories from protein

12% of calories from fat

4 grams of fat

4 grams of fiber

* If you are lactose intolerant, treat the evaporated skimmed milk with lactase enzyme drops, using two times your usual amount or eliminate the evaporated skimmed milk and use all lactose-reduced milk.
** Use lactose-reduced milk if you are lactose intolerant.

Winter Vegetable Soup
SERVES 4

3 cups defatted chicken stock, preferably homemade (see page 208)
2 medium carrots, coarsely chopped
2 small parsnips, coarsely chopped
1 medium onion, coarsely chopped
½ pound celery root, coarsely chopped

*¼ teaspoon freshly ground nutmeg
½ teaspoon salt (omit if you are using canned broth)
1 teaspoon sugar
2 tablespoons chopped fresh dill

1   In 3-quart saucepan, bring stock to boil over medium high heat.
2   Add vegetables, reduce heat to medium low, cover, and simmer for 30 minutes.
3   Remove soup to food processor or blender and puree until smooth. (Do in batches if necessary.)
4   Return to pan. Add spices, heat through, and serve.

Note: This is a thick soup. Add an additional cup of stock if you would prefer a thinner soup. For an interesting variation, add 1 cup of brown rice or barley.

Nutritional information per serving
76 calories
71% of calories from carbohydrate
26% of calories from protein

3% of calories from fat
less than 1 gram of fat
3 grams of fiber

Salmon Mousse
SERVES 4

1 envelope unflavored gelatin
15½ ounce can salmon
**1 cup plain nonfat yogurt
1 small onion, quartered

1 stalk celery, cut in 3 pieces
1 tablespoon lemon juice
1 tablespoon fresh parsley, minced

* Nutmeg is a Flag Food for some people.
** Yogurt is usually well tolerated by lactose intolerant individuals. If you are unable to tolerate yogurt, take 1 lactase enzyme tablet with the mousse.

1 Drain salmon liquid into cup measure. Add enough cold water to equal ⅔ cup.

2 Pour liquid into small saucepan. Sprinkle gelatin on liquid and let it soften for 5 minutes. Heat liquid until gelatin melts.

3 Remove skin from salmon and crush bones. (The bones are included because they are so soft and are an excellent source of calcium.) In blender, puree salmon, yogurt, onion, and celery.

4 In medium bowl, stir together salmon puree, gelatin mixture, lemon juice, and parsley until thoroughly mixed.

5 Place bowl in refrigerator until mousse is partially set.

6 Coat 4-cup mold with nonstick vegetable oil spray. Pour partially gelled mousse into mold. Chill until firm, about 3 hours.

7 Unmold the mousse by inverting onto a platter lined with lettuce leaves. Serve with crackers or cocktail bread.

Nutritional information per serving

200 calories	31% of calories from fat
14% of calories from carbohydrate	7 grams of fat
55% of calories from protein	1 gram of fiber

Tomato Basil Soup

SERVES 4

This soup is best made at the height of tomato and basil season. It freezes well, so can be eaten all winter long when you want the feel of summer.

2½ cups chicken stock, preferably homemade (see page 208)	1 cup fresh basil leaves, cleaned
1 medium yellow onion, chopped	2 teaspoons honey
2 pounds ripe tomatoes (about 4 medium), peeled and quartered	1 bay leaf
	¼ teaspoon salt, or to taste (omit if you are using canned broth)

1 Bring ½ cup of stock to a boil in a 2-quart nonaluminum saucepan. Add onion and cook over medium heat until soft. If extra liquid is necessary, use a small amount of water.

2 Add tomatoes, basil, honey, and bay leaf. Reduce heat to low, cover, and cook for about 10 minutes, stirring occasionally.

3 Puree mixture in blender or food processor. Press through strainer to remove seeds. Return to saucepan.

4 Add remaining 2 cups of stock and salt if desired. Excellent hot or cold!

Nutritional information per serving

99 calories	5% of calories from fat
69% of calories from carbohydrate	less than 1 gram of fat
26% of calories from protein	5 grams of fiber

Turkey Meatball Soup
SERVES 6 TO 8

This soup is very low in sodium if you use homemade chicken stock. You may want to add a teaspoon of salt to the recipe in step 3. Do not add salt if you are using canned chicken broth.

¾ pound ground turkey
1 tablespoon soy sauce, preferably reduced sodium
1 tablespoon dry sherry
1 tablespoon cornstarch
2 tablespoons finely chopped cilantro
2 tablespoons coarsely chopped water chestnuts (about 6)
¼ cup whole wheat breadcrumbs

5 cups defatted chicken stock (see page 208)
3 cups water
1½ cups cooked brown rice
¼ cup sliced water chestnuts (about 12)
3 cups coarsely chopped romaine lettuce or other green
1 tablespoon sesame oil

1 Mix turkey, soy sauce, sherry, cornstarch, cilantro, chopped water chestnuts and breadcrumbs together. Shape into about 20 meatballs.

2 Bring broth and water to boil in large pot. Add meatballs, turn heat to medium, and cook for 5 minutes covered.

3 Add rice, sliced water chestnuts, romaine, and oil. Turn heat down to low. Cover and cook another 10 minutes. Serve hot.

Nutritional information per serving

212 calories	23% of calories from fat
37% of calories from carbohydrate	5 grams of fat
40% of calories from protein	2 grams of fiber

34 *Entrees*
Fish and Seafood

Baked Tomato-Orange Flounder

Fettuccini with Clam Sauce

Flounder in a Flash

Mediterranean Monk Fish

Poached Flounder in Creamy Sauce

Scallops in a Veggie Nest

Snappy Seafood Salad

Sweet and Sour Shrimp

Teriyaki Salmon Kabobs

Tuna Patties

Baked Tomato-Orange Flounder

SERVES 4

Substitute any lean fish of your choice for the flounder. This is a very simple dish, equally suitable for your family or for company.

1 pound flounder filets

SAUCE

¼ cup white wine
1 medium onion, chopped
1 cup canned crushed tomatoes
*¼ cup frozen unsweetened orange
   juice concentrate

3 tablespoons frozen unsweetened
   apple juice concentrate
⅓ cup water
½ teaspoon thyme
slices of orange

* Orange juice may be irritating to the esophagus. Replace with extra apple juice.

1   Preheat oven to 350°.

2   Coat shallow baking pan with nonstick vegetable oil spray. Lay fish filets in pan forming single layer.

3   Pour wine into small saucepan and bring to a boil. Add onion and sauté until transparent.

4   Add tomatoes and simmer 5 minutes.

5   Add orange and apple juice concentrates, water, and thyme and simmer 5 minutes.

6   Pour sauce over fish filets in baking dish and bake for 25 to 30 minutes. Remove to serving platter and garnish with fresh orange slices.

Nutritional information per serving

205 calories	7% of calories from fat
47% of calories from carbohydrate	2 grams of fat
46% of calories from protein	2 grams of fiber

Fettuccini with Clam Sauce

SERVES 4

3 dozen little neck clams	½ cup white wine or dry vermouth
1 yellow bell pepper, cut in thin strips	*½ cup skim milk
3 large shallots, minced	1 teaspoon thyme
1 leek, white part only, chopped	2 tablespoons minced parsley
	12 ounces fettuccini, uncooked

1   Scrub the clams well, discarding any that are open.

2   Combine pepper, shallots, leek, and wine in large heavy skillet with lid. Cover and cook over medium low heat until very tender, about 25 minutes.

3   Transfer mixture to processor or blender. Puree until very smooth (add more wine if necessary). Return the puree to skillet.

4   Stir milk into puree. Boil gently, stirring frequently, about 10 minutes. Add clams and herbs, cover, and let simmer for 5 to 7 minutes. Discard unopened clams.

5   Cook fettuccini in large pot of rapidly boiling water until just tender but still firm to bite. Drain well. Add small amount of sauce to pasta and toss to coat the fettuccini.

6   Divide pasta among 4 plates and top with the remaining sauce.

* If you are lactose intolerant, use lactose-reduced milk.

Nutritional information per serving
- 462 calories
- 67% of calories from carbohydrate
- 27% of calories from protein
- 6% of calories from fat
- 3 grams of fat
- 2 grams of fiber

Flounder in a Flash
SERVES 4

1 large onion, sliced thinly

1 pound flounder filets

SAUCE

*¼ cup plain nonfat or low-fat yogurt
1 tablespoon lemon juice

1 tablespoon Dijon style mustard
1 tablespoon prepared horseradish

1 Coat broiler pan with nonstick vegetable oil spray. Spread sliced onions over bottom of pan. Place fish filets on top of onions in single layer.

2 Mix together sauce ingredients in small bowl. Spread sauce over fish filets.

3 Broil fish for 5 to 10 minutes (depending on thickness). Serve.

Nutritional information per serving
- 130 calories
- 16% of calories from carbohydrate
- 74% of calories from protein
- 10% of calories from fat
- 1 gram of fat
- 1 gram of fiber

Mediterranean Monk Fish
SERVES 4

2 teaspoons olive oil
1½ pounds monk fish
2 teaspoons dried basil

1 tablespoon capers, drained
about 20 black olives, chopped
2 tomatoes, sliced

1 Preheat oven to 350°.

2 Cut square of aluminum foil large enough to hold the monk fish. Brush oil over the foil.

3 Place fish in center of foil. Rub basil into fish. Top with capers, olives, and tomatoes. Form a seal with the aluminum foil.

* Most lactose intolerant individuals can tolerate yogurt without any problem. If you do not, then take 1 lactase enzyme tablet with this meal.

4   Bake fish for about 20 to 25 minutes or until it just flakes. Serve.

Nutritional information per serving

265 calories

5% of calories from carbohydrate

61% of calories from protein

34% of calories from fat

10 grams of fat

1 gram of fiber

Poached Flounder in Creamy Sauce
SERVES 4

This is an incredibly easy recipe and yet rich in flavor.

1 pound flounder filet

1 cup dry vermouth

*1½ cups evaporated skimmed
    milk

¾ teaspoon allspice

1   Place flounder and vermouth in large skillet. Cover and simmer until flounder is cooked, about 8 to 10 minutes.

2   Remove flounder from pan to serving plate and cover to keep warm.

3   Boil cooking liquid until reduced to about ¼ cup. Add evaporated milk and allspice and cook until thickened, stirring continuously.

4   Pour sauce over flounder and serve.

Nutritional information per serving

180 calories

26% of calories from carbohydrate

67% of calories from protein

7% of calories from fat

1 gram of fat

0 grams of fiber

Scallops in a Veggie Nest
SERVES 4

This is a lovely dish to look at and also tastes great. There is a lot of work involved in slicing the vegetables, so you may want to use this as a company meal.

* If you are lactose intolerant, make the evaporated skimmed milk into lactose-free milk by using lactase enzyme drops. Use double the usual amount for 1½ cups of milk and do this 24 hours in advance. Regular low-lactose milk will not work well in this recipe because it is too thin, but if you do try it, use only ¾ cup.

2 medium carrots, cut into matchstick-size julienne strips

2 medium red peppers, cut into matchstick-size julienne strips

1 medium zucchini, skin on, cut into matchstick-size julienne strips

1 cup dry white wine or dry vermouth

4 tablespoons lemon juice

3 green onions, white part only, chopped

¼ cup chopped fresh basil (if unavailable, use 3½ tablespoons of chopped fresh parsley and ½ tablespoon of dried basil)

2 tablespoons chopped fresh dill

2 tablespoons dry sherry

2 teaspoons cornstarch

1 pound bay scallops

1 Prepare vegetables and set aside.

2 Bring wine and lemon juice to a boil in a medium-sized saucepan. Add onions and basil and allow to simmer uncovered at medium heat for about 5 minutes to reduce by half.

3 Meanwhile, steam carrots, peppers, and zucchini about 1½ minutes. Turn heat off, toss with dill, and cover to keep warm.

4 Combine sherry and cornstarch. Add to reduced sauce, stirring. Heat to boiling, add scallops, and cook for 3 to 4 minutes until done, stirring occasionally.

5 Arrange vegetables in a nest on each plate and mound scallops in the middle. Pour a little sauce over each serving. Serve hot.

Nutritional information per serving

166 calories

30% of calories from carbohydrate

60% of calories from protein

10% of calories from fat

2 grams of fat

2 grams of fiber

Snappy Seafood Salad
SERVES 6

DRESSING

*½ cup plain nonfat yogurt

½ cup low-fat mayonnaise

1 tablespoon lemon juice

2 teaspoons Dijon style mustard

2 tablespoons prepared horseradish

* Yogurt is usually well tolerated by lactose intolerant individuals. If you are unable to tolerate yogurt, take 1 lactase enzyme tablet with this meal or replace the yogurt with low-fat mayonnaise. (This will make the salad higher in fat.)

SALAD

1 pound imitation crabmeat or other seafood	2 medium carrots, grated
½ pound green beans, blanched, cut in 1-inch pieces	1 medium onion, chopped

1 In a small bowl combine all dressing ingredients.

2 In a medium bowl, mix together all prepared salad ingredients. Pour the dressing over them and toss.

3 Serve on pita bread or a bed of lettuce.

Variation: Add cooked, cooled pasta to seafood and vegetables and toss with dressing for a main dish pasta salad.

Nutritional information per serving

263 calories	33% of calories from fat
36% of calories from carbohydrate	10 grams of fat
31% of calories from protein	2 grams of fiber

Sweet and Sour Shrimp

SERVES 4

Other types of fish or seafood can be used as substitutes in this recipe. Be prepared—you'll never have leftovers of this tasty dish! Garlic is a great addition to this dish, if you can tolerate it. Add 1 or 2 cloves of finely chopped garlic to the sauce.

SAUCE

¼ cup lemon juice	¼ cup tomato paste
¼ cup soy sauce (preferably reduced sodium)	2 tablespoons honey
	6 tablespoons water

MAIN DISH

1 cup white wine	¾ pound mushrooms, sliced
1½ pounds fresh shrimp, shelled and cleaned	8 ounce can sliced water chestnuts, drained
2 medium green peppers, cut in 1-inch squares	

1 In a medium bowl, whisk together sauce ingredients until thoroughly mixed. Set aside.

2 Pour wine into large skillet. Bring to a simmer; poach shrimp for about 3 minutes. Remove shrimp from skillet with slotted spoon and place in bowl with sauce.

3 Simmer green peppers and mushrooms in remaining wine until tender. Pour off any wine left in skillet.

4 Add sauce, shrimp, and water chestnuts to skillet and cook over medium heat for several minutes until heated through.

5 Serve over rice or noodles.

Nutritional information per serving
 223 calories
 44% of calories from carbohydrate
 49% of calories from protein

 7% of calories from fat
 2 grams of fat
 2 grams of fiber

Teriyaki Salmon Kabobs
SERVES 6

The directions in this recipe are for a broiler, but it would work equally well on a barbecue grill.

MARINADE

2 tablespoons soy sauce, preferably
 reduced sodium
2 tablespoons dry sherry

3 tablespoons unsweetened
 pineapple juice

KABOB

3 pounds fresh salmon steak,
 1 inch thick
3 small zucchini, cut crosswise
 into 8 pieces each

12 cherry tomatoes, whole
12 mushrooms, whole

1 Combine marinade ingredients in small bowl.

2 Remove fish skin and bones. Cut into 1-inch cubes (about 48 pieces). Place in plastic bag with marinade mixture, close bag, and marinate in refrigerator for 1 to 2 hours.

3 While fish is marinating, steam zucchini until crisp but tender.

4 Coat broiler pan with nonstick vegetable oil spray. Alternately thread fish and vegetables onto 12 skewers using 4 pieces of fish, 2 pieces of zucchini, 1 tomato, and 1 mushroom for each kabob. Lay kabobs on broiler pan.

5   Broil about 3 inches from heat, 3 to 5 minutes per side. Be careful not to overcook fish because it will dry out and fall off skewers.

6   Serve on bed of cooked grain, such as rice or barley.

Nutritional information per serving

240 calories	33% of calories from fat
12% of calories from carbohydrate	9 grams of fat
55% of calories from protein	2 grams of fiber

Tuna Patties
SERVES 3

1 medium zucchini, grated and patted dry with paper towel	1 egg or 2 egg whites
6½ ounce can waterpacked tuna, well drained	1 teaspoon lemon juice
	¼ teaspoon cumin
3 slices whole wheat bread, made into bread crumbs in blender	1 tablespoon olive oil

1   Mix zucchini, tuna, and bread crumbs together in medium bowl.

2   Add egg, lemon juice, and cumin. Stir until well mixed.

3   Shape into 3 patties.

4   Heat oil in medium skillet. Cook patties in skillet over medium heat until browned on both sides, about 8 minutes total time.

5   Serve on whole grain roll with lettuce and tomato.

Nutritional information per serving

215 calories	33% of calories from fat
24% of calories from carbohydrate	8 grams of fat
43% of calories from protein	4 grams of fiber

35 *Entrees*
Meat

Beef Kabobs

Beef Stew with Cranberries

Marinated and Grilled Flank Steak

Stir-Fry Orange Beef

Veal with Sun-Dried Tomatoes

Very Veggie Meatloaf

Beef Kabobs
SERVES 4

⅔ cup dry red wine
2 teaspoons sugar
4 teaspoons olive or canola oil
4 teaspoons lemon juice
1 teaspoon basil
1 teaspoon thyme

1 pound lean round steak, cut into
   24 cubes
2 green or red peppers, cut into
   24 squares
1 medium onion, cut into 24 pieces

1 Combine wine, sugar, oil, lemon juice, basil, and thyme in small bowl. Add beef cubes and marinate in refrigerator for several hours or overnight.

2 Remove beef from marinade, reserving marinade.

3 Preheat broiler or grill.

4 Alternately thread meat, peppers, and onions onto 8 skewers, using 3 pieces of each per skewer.

5 Grill or broil about 3 to 4 inches from heat source, basting frequently with reserved marinade. Cook for about 10 minutes or to desired doneness. Serve 2 kabobs per person on a bed of brown rice.

Nutritional information per serving

245 calories

14% calories from carbohydrate

48% calories from protein

38% calories from fat

10 grams of fat

1 gram of fiber

Beef Stew with Cranberries
SERVES 6

While this is an unlikely combination, it works well and is a very interesting beef stew. It's wonderful on a cold January day!

2 pounds lean stew meat, trimmed of all visible fat and cut into 1-inch cubes

1½–2 cups burgundy wine

2–3 small cinnamon sticks

½ teaspoon lightly crushed coriander seeds

1 large onion, sliced

2 tablespoons red wine vinegar

1 tablespoon tomato paste

½ teaspoon salt, if desired

2 tablespoons whole wheat flour

1 tablespoon honey

1 cup fresh cranberries, washed and finely chopped (most easily done in a food processor or blender)

1 Marinate beef in mixture of 1½ cups wine, cinnamon sticks, and coriander all day or overnight. Drain beef, reserving marinade and spices. Add enough extra wine to reserved marinade to total 2 cups.

2 Set heavy 6-quart pot over medium heat. Add meat in batches and cook over medium heat until brown. It is not necessary to add oil. Transfer to plate as each batch is browned.

3 Return meat to pan. Add onion, vinegar, tomato paste, salt, and reserved marinade.

4 Bring to a boil, cover, reduce heat, and simmer slowly for about 1½ hours.

5 Remove ½ cup of sauce and stir into flour until smooth. Return flour mixture to pot. Add honey and cranberries to beef mixture.

6 Increase heat to medium and cook uncovered for 15 additional minutes, stirring frequently.

7 Serve over noodles or rice. (This stew is especially good if refrigerated and reheated the following day. It gives the flavors a chance to blend.)

Nutritional information per serving

292 calories

20% of calories from carbohydrate

55% of calories from protein

25% of calories from fat

8 grams of fat

2 grams of fiber

Marinated and Grilled Flank Steak

SERVES 4

1 pound flank steak, trimmed of all
fat

MARINADE

1 can beer (12 ounces)

2 tablespoons Worcestershire
sauce

1 tablespoon brown sugar

¼ cup chopped parsley

½ teaspoon dried tarragon

½ teaspoon dried thyme

2 bay leaves

2 green onions, white and green
parts, chopped

2 tablespoons red wine vinegar

1 Mix marinade ingredients together and pour over flank steak. Marinate overnight in large sealable plastic bag in refrigerator.

2 Remove steak from marinade. Preheat broiler or grill. Place steak in broiler pan and broil 6 minutes on each side. (Or grill the steak.)

3 Meanwhile, bring marinade to a boil, turn heat to low, and allow to simmer while steak cooks.

4 Carve meat across the grain in paper-thin slices. Spoon some of the sauce over it and pass the remaining sauce separately.

Nutritional information per serving

183 calories

12% of calories from carbohydrate

61% of calories from protein

27% of calories from fat

5 grams of fat

less than 1 gram of fiber

Stir-Fry Orange Beef

SERVES 4

The entire cooking process for this stir-fry takes under 5 minutes. If your vegetables are all set to go, it's a quick delicious meal.

1 pound flank steak, trimmed of fat
*⅔ cup orange juice concentrate
1 tablespoon lime juice
**2 tablespoons mirin
2 tablespoons reduced-sodium soy sauce
½ tablespoon minced fresh ginger
¼ cup dry vermouth

2 teaspoons cornstarch
½ pound carrots, sliced
½ pound snow peas, strings removed
8 ounce can sliced water chestnuts, drained
3 green onions, chopped

1 Slice flank steak across the grain into thin strips. (It is easier to do this if you put the flank steak in the freezer for a little while before slicing.) Place into large sealable plastic bag.

2 Mix together juices, mirin, soy sauce, ginger, and vermouth. Pour over beef, and marinate overnight.

3 Drain meat, reserving marinade. Whisk cornstarch into marinade.

4 Heat wok or large nonstick skillet over high heat. Add beef and cook for 1 to 1½ minutes to desired doneness. Remove to platter.

5 Add carrots and cook for about 30 seconds, stirring constantly. Add snow peas and water chestnuts, cook for an additional 15 to 30 seconds.

6 Return beef to pan and add marinade-cornstarch mixture. Bring to a boil and cook for about 1 minute or until sauce is desired thickness. Add green onions, remove from heat, and serve over rice or another grain of your choice.

Nutritional information per serving

312 calories
40% of calories from carbohydrate
42% of calories from protein

18% of calories from fat
6 grams of fat
6 grams of fiber

---

* Orange juice can be irritating to the esophagus. It really is essential to this recipe, so there is no replacement.
** Mirin is a sweet rice wine available in oriental markets. It will keep in your refrigerator indefinitely, so buy a bottle to have on hand.

Veal with Sun-Dried Tomatoes

SERVES 4

½ cup sun-dried tomatoes
1 tablespoon olive oil
4 veal scallopini (1 pound total
   weight)
½ cup dry white wine or vermouth
½ cup sliced mushrooms

⅓ cup chopped shallots
1 teaspoon lemon juice
2 teaspoons fresh parsley, chopped
2 teaspoons fresh basil, chopped
   (½ teaspoon dried)
salt to taste

1 Soak sun-dried tomatoes in hot water for at least 10 minutes. Drain and slice into strips.

2 Heat oil in large skillet and quickly sauté the veal, about 1 minute on each side. Remove and drain on paper towels.

3 Add wine, mushrooms, tomatoes, and shallots to the skillet. Sauté until vegetables are tender. Sprinkle lemon juice, parsley, and basil over softened vegetables and stir.

4 Add veal to the sauce to reheat. Season with salt if desired.

Nutritional information per serving
260 calories
12% of calories from carbohydrate
41% of calories from protein

47% of calories from fat
13 grams of fat
2 grams of fiber

Very Veggie Meatloaf

SERVES 6

This is a tasty meatloaf as heavy on the vegetables as on the meat. It is good either plain with a marinara sauce (see page 286) or as a sandwich filler.

½ pound potato, peeled and
   shredded
½ pound onion (1 medium),
   shredded
¼ pound carrot (1 large), shredded
¼ cup chopped parsley
2 tablespoons white wine
   Worcestershire sauce

¼ cup breadcrumbs, preferably
   whole wheat
1 egg white
1 tablespoon Dijon style mustard
½ teaspoon dried oregano
½ teaspoon dried basil
1 pound lean ground beef

1 Preheat oven to 350°.
2 In large bowl, mix together all ingredients.
3 Press mixture into loaf pan. Bake for 1 hour.

Nutritional information per serving

240 calories   40% of calories from fat
29% of calories from carbohydrate   11 grams of fat
31% of calories from protein   2 grams of fiber

36 *Entrees*
Meatless

Eggless Salad

Spinach Rice Casserole

Stuffed Bell Peppers

Tofu Stroganoff

Eggless Salad
SERVES 4

This is very similar to egg salad, but it is lower in fat and is cholesterol-free. Although this recipe appears to be high in fat, it is much lower than a mayonnaise-based egg salad

SALAD

⅔ pound firm tofu, cut in ½-inch cubes

½ large green pepper, diced

1 large stalk celery, diced

1 large carrot, grated

½ medium red onion, diced

*¼ cup sunflower seeds, toasted

DRESSING

⅓ pound firm tofu

2 tablespoons prepared mustard

soy sauce to taste

1 Prepare all salad ingredients as described.
2 Blend together dressing ingredients in blender or food processor.

---

* Seeds can be gas producing. You may be able to tolerate this small amount, but if not you may omit them. This will decrease the fat content as well.

3   Stir salad and dressing together gently until well mixed.

4   Serve eggless salad on bread or bed of greens. It is especially good served on whole wheat pita bread and topped with alfalfa sprouts.

Nutritional information per serving

240 calories	52% of calories from fat
16% of calories from carbohydrate	15 grams of fat
32% of calories from protein	1 gram of fiber

Spinach Rice Casserole

SERVES 4

Leftovers of this main dish casserole are good cold for lunch.

1 egg (or 2 egg whites)	2 cups mushrooms, quartered
*2 cups 1% low-fat cottage cheese	1 medium onion chopped
3 cups cooked brown rice	1 teaspoon marjoram
4 cups fresh spinach, torn, uncooked, well drained	**2 tablespoons grated Romano cheese

1   Preheat oven to 375°.

2   Beat egg and cottage cheese together.

3   Stir in rice, spinach, mushrooms, onion, and marjoram until well blended.

4   Pour mixture into 9 x 13-inch baking dish that has been coated with nonstick vegetable oil spray. Sprinkle with grated cheese.

5   Bake for 30 minutes.

Nutritional information per serving

320 calories	11% of calories from fat
60% of calories from carbohydrate	4 grams of fat
29% of calories from protein	8 grams of fiber

---

* If you have a lactose intolerance, look for low-lactose cottage cheese or take 2 lactase enzyme tablets with this meal.

** This small amount of Romano cheese should be well tolerated in all but the most severely lactose intolerant individuals. The cheese can be left off for those individuals.

Stuffed Bell Peppers

SERVES 4

4 large bell peppers
* ½ cup dry bulgur wheat
3 tablespoons chopped onion
1 tablespoon vegetable oil, preferably olive or canola
½ pound tofu, cut into small cubes
1½ cups tomato puree
2 tablespoons green pepper, finely chopped

2 tablespoons celery, finely chopped
1 tablespoon brown sugar
1 tablespoon oregano
¼ teaspoon allspice
¼ teaspoon cloves (optional)
1 cup *cooked* brown rice
1 tablespoon grated carrots

1 Preheat oven to 350°.

2 Wash and core peppers. Steam for 20 minutes.

3 Soak bulgur in ⅓ cup warm water. Set aside.

4 In large skillet, sauté onion in oil until softened.

5 Add tofu. Stir until evenly browned.

6 Add 1 cup of tomato puree, diced green pepper, celery, brown sugar, herbs, and spices. Heat mixture until bubbly. Reduce heat to a simmer and cook for about 15 minutes.

7 Add rice and bulgur. Stir.

8 Fill each pepper with stuffing.

9 Place in casserole and top with the reserved ½ cup tomato puree. Pour about ¼ inch water in bottom of pan.

10 Bake for 30 minutes. Remove from oven and sprinkle grated carrots on top of stuffed peppers.

Nutritional information per serving

297 calories
66% of calories from carbohydrate
13% of calories from protein

21% of calories from fat
7 grams of fat
4 grams of fiber

Tofu Stroganoff

SERVES 4

Try this delicious lower fat version of a classic main dish!

* Bulgur wheat is available in health food or bulk food stores.

MARINADE

1 pound firm tofu
¼ cup soy sauce, preferably low sodium

*½ teaspoon garlic powder
*⅛ teaspoon black pepper
⅛ teaspoon cumin

MAIN DISH

1 tablespoon cornstarch
**1 cup plain nonfat yogurt
1 teaspoon olive oil
1 medium onion, minced
½ pound mushrooms, sliced

½ teaspoon basil
*dash nutmeg
4 cups uncooked flat noodles
¼ cup white wine

1 At least 3 hours prior to meal, begin marinating tofu; it can be marinated overnight. Cut tofu into ½-inch cubes and place in small deep bowl. Add soy sauce, spices, and enough water to cover. Mix well and put into refrigerator until ready to prepare main dish.

2 Begin heating water to cook noodles in large pot. Drain tofu of marinade. Whisk cornstarch into yogurt.

3 Heat oil in large nonstick frying pan. Cook onion in oil for 2 to 3 minutes, add tofu and mushrooms, and cook 2 to 3 minutes more. Add basil and nutmeg. Reduce heat, cover, and cook about 10 minutes. Begin cooking noodles.

4 When mushrooms are tender, add wine and yogurt-cornstarch mixture. Heat through over low heat. When noodles are done, drain in colander.

5 Serve stroganoff over noodles.

Nutritional information per serving
550 calories
52% of calories from carbohydrate
25% of calories from protein

23% of calories from fat
14 grams of fat
4 grams of fiber

---

* Garlic powder, black pepper, and nutmeg are gastric irritants. You may omit them if you are unable to tolerate them.
** Yogurt is usually well tolerated by lactose intolerant individuals. If you are unable to tolerate yogurt, take 1 lactase enzyme tablet with this meal.

37 *Entrees*
Poultry

Chicken and Herbs Baked in Foil
SERVES 4

4 chicken breast halves, boned and skinned
1 teaspoon olive oil
¼ cup chopped fresh dill

*¼ cup chopped fresh mint
4 scallions, diced
1 lemon, thinly sliced

1 Preheat oven to 350°.
2 Brush each chicken breast with ¼ teaspoon of olive oil. Place each breast on a large piece of aluminum foil.

---

* Mint commonly causes gastric distress and heartburn. If you are unable to tolerate mint, replace it with fresh coriander (also called cilantro or Chinese parsley).

3 Mix together dill, mint, and scallions. Divide mixture and spread equally over chicken breasts.

4 Top each breast with 2 to 3 lemon slices. Fold foil over, making a tight seal.

5 Bake for 30 minutes. Remove from foil and serve.

Nutritional information per serving

230 calories

7% of calories from carbohydrate

70% of calories from protein

23% of calories from fat

6 grams of fat

less than 1 gram of fiber

Chicken Breasts in Creamy Mustard Sauce
SERVES 4

4 chicken breast halves, each about 6 ounces, skinned, boned, trimmed

3 tablespoons flour, preferably whole wheat

½ teaspoon dried marjoram

½ teaspoon dried thyme

*½ teaspoon fresh ground black pepper

1 teaspoon butter or margarine

½ cup dry vermouth or white wine

1 cup defatted chicken stock, preferably homemade (see page 210)

2 tablespoons Dijon style mustard

**¼ cup evaporated skimmed milk

Fresh thyme sprigs

1 Pound chicken breasts between sheets of waxed paper to the thickness of ¼ inch.

2 Combine flour, herbs, and spices. Transfer 1 tablespoon of mixture to small bowl and reserve. Rub remainder into chicken.

3 Coat skillet with nonstick vegetable oil spray. Add butter and melt. Add chicken and cook until brown, about 2 minutes per side. Transfer to plate.

4 Add vermouth to skillet and boil until reduced to a glaze, scraping up any browned bits, about 1 minute. Mix in stock and mustard and boil for 2 to 3 minutes.

5 Mix evaporated skimmed milk into reserved flour. Whisk in ¼ cup of the hot stock/mustard mixture and return to pan. Simmer until thickened and smooth, stirring constantly for about 3 minutes.

---

* Black pepper is a gastric irritant. If you are unable to tolerate it, replace the black pepper with ½ teaspoon of chervil.

** A lactose intolerant individual should be able to tolerate the small amount of lactose in one serving. However, if you are severely lactose intolerant, either treat the evaporated skimmed milk with lactase enzyme drops (use two times your usual amount) or take 1 lactase enzyme tablet with this meal.

6 Return chicken to skillet and cook at medium low heat until opaque, about 1 minute per side.

7 Serve chicken with extra sauce on the side. Garnish with fresh thyme sprigs.

Nutritional information per serving

290 calories	21% of calories from fat
11% of calories from carbohydrate	7 grams of fat
68% of calories from protein	0 grams of fiber

Chicken Fajitas
SERVES 4

2 whole chicken breasts, boned and skinned	4 scallions, coarsely chopped
*1 cup tomato juice	1 bunch cilantro, chopped
2 tablespoons lime juice	1 red or green bell pepper, coarsely chopped
1 tablespoon reduced-sodium soy sauce	8 flour tortillas
2 tomatoes, coarsely chopped	1 cup mock sour cream (see page 287)

1 Cut the chicken across the grain into thin strips. It is easier to do this if the chicken is slightly frozen. Place the chicken in a nonaluminum bowl.

2 Pour tomato juice, lime juice, and soy sauce over chicken strips and allow to marinate several hours or overnight. (If you can tolerate it, 2 cloves of finely chopped garlic is a great addition to the marinade.)

3 Meanwhile, prepare tomatoes, scallions, cilantro, and pepper. Arrange on serving platter and refrigerate.

4 Preheat broiler. Drain marinade from chicken. Place marinade in small, nonaluminum saucepan, bring to a boil, and allow to simmer while chicken is cooking.

5 Broil chicken strips in a single layer, 4 inches from heat source, for about 3 to 5 minutes or until done. Turn for the last minute of cooking.

6 Seal tortillas in aluminum foil and place in bottom of oven to heat while you broil the chicken (or place in 350° oven for 5 to 10 minutes).

7 To serve, place chicken strips, vegetables, and marinade sauce (if desired) in center of tortilla. Top with mock sour cream. Roll or fold tortilla and eat as a sandwich.

* Tomato juice can be irritating to the esophagus. It can be replaced with chicken stock.

Nutritional information per serving

450 calories	17% of calories from fat
39% of calories from carbohydrate	9 grams of fat
44% of calories from protein	2 grams of fiber

Chicken-Vegetable Stir-Fry

SERVES 4

½ cup defatted chicken stock or broth (see page 208)

1 whole chicken breast (10 to 12 ounces), boned, skinned, and cut into bite-sized pieces

MARINADE

¼ cup dry white wine

¼ cup reduced-sodium soy sauce

8 ounce can of sliced or chunk pineapple (undrained) in its own juice, pureed

*2 garlic cloves, finely minced

1 teaspoon fresh ginger, finely minced

VEGETABLES

**1 bunch broccoli, stalks peeled and sliced on diagonal; florets cut into bite-size pieces

¼ pound snow peas, strings removed

2 red peppers, cut into julienne strips

1 yellow pepper, cut into julienne strips

2 teaspoons cornstarch

½ teaspoon vegetable oil, preferably canola or olive oil

½ pound whole wheat pasta twists

1 Heat chicken stock to boiling in small skillet. Add chicken pieces and poach until done, about 4 to 5 minutes.

2 Combine marinade ingredients. Add chicken and cooking broth and marinate overnight in refrigerator.

3 Heat 2 to 3 quarts of water for pasta.

4 Prepare vegetables.

5 Remove chicken from marinade, reserving marinade.

6 Remove ½ cup of marinade and mix with cornstarch. Set aside.

7 Put oil into wok or large skillet and spread it with a paper towel. Heat wok.

---

* Garlic is gas producing. If you are unable to tolerate the garlic, it may be omitted.
** Broccoli is gas producing. Substitute ½ pound of green beans if you are unable to tolerate the broccoli.

8 Put pasta into boiling water. Cook until done (about 7 minutes), stirring as necessary, while you stir-fry the vegetables.

9 Add broccoli to wok and stir-fry for about 2 minutes. Add snow peas and stir-fry for about 1 minute. Add pepper and stir-fry for about 30 seconds. Add chicken for another 30 seconds. If additional liquid is necessary, add a small amount of reserved marinade.

10 Remove vegetable-chicken mixture to large bowl or platter. Add the reserved marinade to wok and bring to a boil. Add the cornstarch-marinade mixture and stir until it reaches the desired thickness.

11 Return the chicken-vegetable mixture to the wok and heat through.

12 Meanwhile, drain the pasta.

13 Serve chicken-vegetable mixture over pasta.

Nutritional information per serving

423 calories

52% of calories from carbohydrate

37% of calories from protein

11% of calories from fat

5 grams of fat

8 grams of fiber

Chicken with Mushrooms and Sun-dried Tomatoes
SERVES 4

This is a wonderful company meal, yet so simple you'll want to prepare it for your family.

1 cup chicken stock, preferably homemade (see page 208)

½ cup dry sherry

2 whole chicken breasts, skinned, boned, and split

¾ pound mushrooms, sliced

⅓ cup finely chopped onion

⅓ cup chopped parsley

2 ounces sun-dried tomatoes (12 to 15), soaked in 2 cups of boiling water for 5 minutes, drained and chopped. Reserve ½ cup of soaking liquid.

½ teaspoon dried basil

2 teaspoons Dijon style mustard

Fresh basil sprigs

1 Bring ½ cup of chicken stock and sherry to a boil in large skillet. Add chicken and cook for about 15 seconds on each side. Add mushrooms, onion, and parsley, turn heat to low, cover, and simmer for about 5 minutes or until chicken is cooked through. Remove chicken to platter.

2 Add remaining ½ cup of chicken stock, tomatoes, ½ cup of reserved tomato liquid, basil, and mustard. Bring to a boil and cook for 5 to 8 minutes or until liquid is almost completely reduced.

3 Spread mushroom-tomato mixture over a serving platter and place chicken on top. Garnish with fresh basil sprigs.

Nutritional information per serving
275 calories

18% of calories from carbohydrate

65% of calories from protein

17% of calories from fat

5 grams of fat

4 grams of fiber

Creole Topped Potato
SERVES 4

This is a wonderful main dish potato.

4 medium-sized baking potatoes, well scrubbed and dried

2 teaspoons vegetable oil, preferably olive or canola oil

¼ cup chopped onion

½ cup chopped green pepper

½ pound ground turkey

⅛ teaspoon dried basil

1 tablespoon white wine or dry vermouth

½ cup tomato puree

*4 ounces grated cheddar cheese

1 Preheat oven to 375°.

2 Pierce potatoes with fork tines. Wrap in foil and bake 1 hour.

3 While potatoes are baking, heat oil in large pot. Add onion and green pepper and cook until tender, about 10 minutes, stirring often. If additional liquid is necessary use wine or vermouth.

4 Add ground turkey and cook until no longer pink.

5 Add basil, wine, and tomato puree. Bring to boil, lower heat, and simmer covered for 30 minutes.

6 Remove potatoes from oven, unwrap and slice lengthwise. Top each potato half with about ¼ cup of creole mixture and ½ ounce of cheese. Serve.

Nutritional information per serving
453 calories

49% of calories from carbohydrate

24% of calories from protein

27% of calories from fat

14 grams of fat

5 grams of fiber

* You may tolerate a small amount of cheese if you are lactose intolerant, but if not, the cheese may be omitted, or you may take 1 lactase enzyme tablet.

Fruited Chicken Salad

SERVES 4

The grapenuts in this recipe provide an interesting and low-fat alternative to nuts.

2 cups cooked chicken, cubed	½ cup low-fat mayonnaise
2 medium oranges, each section cut into 3 or 4 pieces	1 tablespoon honey
½ cup diced celery	1 tablespoon Dijon style mustard
*½ cup plain nonfat yogurt	½ cup grapenuts cereal
	Salad greens

1 Stir together chicken, oranges, and celery in medium-size bowl.

2 In small bowl, mix together yogurt, mayonnaise, honey, and mustard until well blended.

3 Pour yogurt dressing over chicken salad and toss until well mixed.

4 Just before serving, stir in grapenuts.

5 Serve on a bed of greens. Especially tasty served on a bed of fresh spinach leaves.

Nutritional information per serving

305 calories	31% of calories from fat
37% of calories from carbohydrate	11 grams of fat
32% of calories from protein	2 grams of fiber

Ground Turkey in Zucchini Shells

SERVES 4

4 medium zucchini	1 egg or 2 egg whites
½ pound ground turkey	½ teaspoon thyme
1 medium onion, chopped	**¼ cup grated Romano cheese
½ cup bread crumbs (preferably whole wheat)	

* Most lactose intolerant individuals can tolerate yogurt without any problem. If you do not, you may take 1 lactase enzyme tablet with this meal or use all low-fat mayonnaise. The use of low-fat mayonnaise will increase the fat content of this recipe.

** This small amount of cheese should be tolerated by all but the most severely lactose intolerant individual. If you are unable to tolerate the cheese, take 1 lactase enzyme tablet with this meal.

1 Preheat oven to 350°.

2 Boil whole zucchini until just tender, about 8 minutes.

3 While zucchini are boiling, cook ground turkey and onion in skillet. To prevent sticking, put turkey in cold skillet and begin cooking over low heat. After turkey is cooked, remove from heat and drain off liquid.

4 Cut cooked zucchini in half lengthwise. Scoop out pulp and mash it with a fork. Reserve zucchini shells.

5 Stir mashed zucchini pulp, bread crumbs, egg, and thyme into turkey mixture. Mix well.

6 Spoon mixture evenly into zucchini shells. Sprinkle with grated cheese.

7 Place shells in baking dish and bake in 350° oven for 25 to 30 minutes.

Nutritional information per serving

235 calories	26% of calories from fat
33% of calories from carbohydrate	7 grams of fat
41% of calories from protein	3 grams of fiber

Lemonade Chicken

SERVES 4

3 pounds chicken pieces, skinned	¼ cup reduced-sodium soy sauce
*¾ cup (6 ounces) lemonade concentrate, defrosted	¼ teaspoon ground ginger

1 Skin chicken and place in glass ovenproof pan.

2 Mix lemonade, soy sauce, and ginger together. Pour over chicken. Marinate all day or overnight. Remove chicken from marinade.

3 Preheat broiler. Broil about 5 inches from heat source, about 15 minutes per side. Baste chicken often (about 10 times total while cooking). Serve.

*Nutritional information per serving***

340 calories	37% of calories from fat
14% of calories from carbohydrate	14 grams of fat
49% of calories from protein	0 grams of fiber

---

* Lemonade can be irritating to the esophagus.

** The nutrient analysis was done using chicken thighs and legs. The calorie and fat content would be lowered by using white meat (i.e., breast meat).

Marinated and Grilled Chicken Breast

SERVES 4

You'll find this to be a little different from the typical grilled chicken. It's a quick summer meal that can be prepared outside on the grill, but works just as well under your broiler.

2 whole chicken breasts, boned,
  skinned, and split

MARINADE

4 tablespoons reduced-sodium soy
  sauce
2 tablespoons brown sugar

4 tablespoons dry vermouth
2 tablespoons white wine
  Worcestershire sauce

BASTING SAUCE

½ cup apricot preserves
¼ cup white vinegar

1 tablespoon white wine
  Worcestershire sauce

1   Mix marinade ingredients together in glass bowl or large sealable plastic bag. Add chicken breasts and marinate overnight.

2   In small saucepan, bring basting sauce ingredients to a boil. Turn heat to low and simmer uncovered, stirring occasionally, for 3 minutes.

3   Preheat broiler or grill. Coat broiler pan with nonstick vegetable oil spray. Remove chicken from marinade and discard marinade.

4   Broil or grill 4 inches from heat, basting at least 3 times on each side. Cook for about 5 to 6 minutes per side or until cooked through. Serve immediately.

Nutritional information per serving
336 calories
39% of calories from carbohydrate
49% of calories from protein

12% of calories from fat
5 grams of fat
0 grams of fiber

Oriental Barbecued Chicken

SERVES 4

This is excellent hot, but even better cold for picnics.

3 pounds chicken pieces with skin
  and fat removed

MARINADE

*2 garlic cloves, peeled and finely chopped

½ inch slice ginger, peeled and minced

3 scallions, white and green parts, chopped

2 tablespoons hoisin sauce

2 tablespoons catsup

2 tablespoons reduced-sodium soy sauce

3 tablespoons rice wine vinegar

1 Place chicken in 11 × 8-inch glass baking pan. Mix all ingredients for marinade together and pour over chicken. Cover with aluminum foil. Marinate overnight in refrigerator. Turn chicken over once.

2 Preheat oven to 450°. Bake covered for 20 minutes, basting as necessary. Turn oven down to 350°, turn chicken, baste well. Cook another 20 minutes, basting as necessary.

Nutritional information per serving **

256 calories

9% of calories from carbohydrate

55% of calories from protein

36% of calories from fat

10 grams of fat

0 grams of fiber

* Garlic is gas producing. Omit the garlic if you are unable to tolerate it.
** To decrease the fat content further, use only chicken breasts. This recipe was analyzed using breasts, thighs, and legs. The dark meat of poultry is higher in fat than white meat.

38 *Side Dishes*
Grains and Starches

Barley Delight

Beautiful Bow Tie Pasta

Cinnamon Rice

Cold Barley Salad

Cold Bulgur Wheat Salad

Italian-style Couscous

Kasha and Corn

Rice Salad

Wheat Berry Salad

Whole Grain Pasta Salad

Barley Delight
SERVES 4

3 cups water
1 cup barley
*½ cup raisins

**½ cup plain nonfat yogurt
*¼ teaspoon nutmeg
***¼ cup sesame seeds, toasted

* Raisins are gas producing. You could replace the raisins with dried currants or another dried fruit of your choice. If you are unable to tolerate nutmeg, it can be replaced with cinnamon.
** Yogurt is usually well tolerated by lactose intolerant individuals. Take 1 lactase enzyme tablet with this meal if you are unable to tolerate yogurt.
*** Seeds are gas producing. Omit the seeds if you are unable to tolerate them, although they may be well tolerated in this small amount.

1   Bring 3 cups water and 1 cup barley to a boil. Reduce heat to a simmer, cover, and cook for 35 to 40 minutes or until water is absorbed.

2   Stir in raisins, yogurt, and nutmeg. Mix well.

3   Sprinkle with sesame seeds just before serving.

Nutritional information per serving

296 calories	14% of calories from fat
76% of calories from carbohydrate	5 grams of fat
10% of calories from protein	3 grams of fiber

Beautiful Bow Tie Pasta

SERVES 6

16 ounces bow tie pasta, cooked al dente

2 tablespoons olive oil

½ cup wine vinegar

*½ cup crumbled feta cheese (about 4 ounces)

1 cup snow peas, cleaned and cut in half lengthwise, blanched for 1 minute

1 large sweet red pepper, julienned, blanched for 1 minute

1 large yellow pepper, julienned, blanched for 1 minute

1 carrot cut into coins, blanched for 2 minutes

½ large purple onion, cut into rings, blanched for 2 minutes

1 large red tomato, diced

¼ cup finely chopped parsley

¼ cup coarsely chopped fresh basil

** fresh black pepper

1   Cook pasta al dente, drain, and run under cold water.

2   In small bowl combine the oil, vinegar, and feta cheese and whisk briskly.

3   Combine pasta, vegetables, herbs, and dressing in large bowl and toss gently until all are combined. Top with freshly grated black pepper.

Nutritional information per serving

400 calories	22% of calories from fat
64% of calories from carbohydrate	10 grams of fat
14% of calories from protein	4 grams of fiber

---

* Many people with a lactose intolerance are able to tolerate small amounts of cheese. If you are unable to tolerate the feta cheese, take 1 lactase enzyme tablet with this meal or omit the cheese and use 4 tablespoons of olive oil.

** Omit the black pepper if you find it to be a gastric irritant. (Most people will need to omit it.)

Cinnamon Rice

SERVES 6

This is a very simple yet interesting variation on rice. Try to use brown rice as it is significantly higher in fiber.

2 cups raw brown rice	2 cinnamon sticks
6 cups water	1 tablespoon lemon juice

1 Mix all ingredients together in 3-quart saucepan and bring to a boil.

2 Reduce heat to low, cover, and cook until all the liquid is absorbed, about 45 minutes.

Nutritional information per serving

232 calories	5% of calories from fat
87% of calories from carbohydrate	1 gram of fat
8% of calories from protein	6 grams of fiber

Cold Barley Salad

SERVES 6

1 cup raw barley	1½ tablespoons olive oil
1½ cups chicken stock, preferably homemade (see page 208)	3 stalks celery, diced
1½ cups water	3 small carrots, sliced thinly
3 tablespoons balsamic vinegar	*1 medium red onion, diced

1 Cook barley in broth and water until barley is tender and liquid is absorbed.

2 Stir vinegar and olive oil into hot barley. Chill until serving time.

3 Stir celery, carrot, and onion into cooled barley and serve.

Nutritional information per serving

182 calories	20% of calories from fat
70% of calories from carbohydrate	4 grams of fat
10% of calories from protein	3 grams of fiber

---

* If you are unable to tolerate raw onion, omit it. Try scallions if you tolerate them better.

Cold Bulgur Wheat Salad
SERVES 4

2 cups water, boiling
*1 cup bulgur wheat, dry
1 cucumber, peeled and diced
1 tomato, diced
6 scallions, chopped

1 cup fresh parsley, chopped
4 tablespoons lemon juice
1 tablespoon soy sauce
1 tablespoon olive oil

1   Pour boiling water over bulgur. Soak for 1 hour. Drain off any excess water.
2   Stir remaining ingredients into bulgur and chill until serving.

Nutritional information per serving

216 calories
74% of calories from carbohydrate
10% of calories from protein

16% of calories from fat
4 grams of fat
3 grams of fiber

Italian-Style Couscous
SERVES 4

1 cup sliced mushrooms
½ cup dry white wine or dry
  vermouth
1 teaspoon dried basil

½ cup water
1 tomato, peeled and chopped
**1 cup whole wheat couscous, dry

1   Marinate mushrooms in wine for 30 minutes.
2   Add basil and cook mushrooms in marinade until tender.
3   Add water and tomato and bring to boil. Remove from heat, stir in couscous, cover, and let stand for 5 minutes. Serve.

Nutritional information per serving

168 calories
86% of calories from carbohydrate
10% of calories from protein

4% of calories from fat
less than 1 gram of fat
2 grams of fiber

* Bulgur wheat is a cracked wheat that has been steamed, dried, and cracked into small pieces. It is available in health food stores, bulk food stores, and specialty food stores.
** Couscous is available in health food or bulk food stores. Look for whole wheat couscous, which is higher in fiber. Couscous is finely cracked wheat that has been steamed and dried. Its quick cooking time (5 minutes) makes it a great alternative to rice and other grains.

Kasha and Corn

SERVES 4

1 cup kasha (buckwheat)
1 medium onion, chopped
1 tablespoon olive oil
2 cups chicken stock, preferably
   homemade (see page 208)

*1 cup corn, whole kernel
¼ cup fresh parsley, chopped

1   Sauté kasha and onion in oil until onion is translucent.
2   Add stock and bring to a boil. Cover and simmer until kasha is tender, about 15 minutes.
3   Stir in corn and parsley, heat through, and serve.

Nutritional information per serving
   183 calories
   60% of calories from carbohydrate
   15% of calories from protein

25% of calories from fat
5 grams of fat
4 grams of fiber

Rice Salad

SERVES 4

Although this salad may appear to be high in fat, it contains much less oil than you typically find in a salad. The usual proportion of oil to vinegar in a dressing is 3 parts oil to 1 part vinegar.

SALAD

3 cups cooked brown rice, cooled
1 cup cooked wild rice, cooled
1 large green pepper, sliced

2 medium carrots, scraped and
   sliced on diagonal
¼ cup parsley, chopped

DRESSING

5 tablespoons red wine vinegar
3 tablespoons olive oil
2 teaspoons Dijon style mustard

¼ teaspoon dried tarragon
pinch of basil
pinch of thyme

1   Combine salad ingredients in large serving bowl.
2   Whisk ingredients for dressing together. Pour over salad. Refrigerate several hours before serving.

* Corn can be gas producing. If you are unable to tolerate corn, replace it with green peas.

Nutritional information per serving

302 calories
60% of calories from carbohydrate
7% of calories from protein

33% of calories from fat
11 grams of fat
8 grams of fiber

Wheat Berry Salad
SERVES 4

1½ cups water
*½ cup hard wheat berries (often called winter wheat)
1 cinnamon stick
1 celery stalk, diced
1 medium apple, cored and coarsely chopped, skin on

**¼ cup raisins
½ teaspoon vanilla
½ teaspoon ground coriander
***¼ cup plain low-fat or nonfat yogurt

1 Bring water to a boil. Add wheat berries and cinnamon stick and return to boil. Reduce heat to simmer, cover, and cook about 2 hours or until berries are tender. Drain if necessary and cool.

2 Add celery, apple, raisins, spices, and yogurt. Stir to combine. Refrigerate until ready to serve. Leave cinnamon stick in salad until ready to serve, but remove before serving.

Nutritional information per serving

195 calories
86% of calories from carbohydrate
10% of calories from protein

4% of calories from fat
1 gram of fat
7 grams of fiber

* Wheat berries can be found in health food and bulk food stores. They are delicious and worth the effort to find them and to cook them. Cook extra and freeze them for future use.
** Raisins are gas producing. Omit them if you are unable to tolerate them.
*** Lactose intolerant individuals can usually tolerate yogurt. This is a very small amount per portion and should not cause any problems. If you would prefer, you may use low-fat mayonnaise.

Whole Grain Pasta Salad

SERVES 6

*1 cup broccoli flowerets
¾ cup carrots, sliced into coins
1 small zucchini, unpeeled, cut into 1-inch chunks
½ cup mushrooms, halved

1¼ cups cherry tomatoes, halved
1¼ cups whole wheat pasta, preferably corkscrew, cooked al dente (about 3 cups cooked)

DRESSING

**½ cup plain low-fat yogurt
¼ cup red wine vinegar
***2 tablespoons grated Parmesan cheese

1 tablespoon low-fat mayonnaise
1 tablespoon parsley

1 Place broccoli and carrots in a vegetable steamer and steam for 5 minutes. Add zucchini and steam for 3 more minutes.

2 Combine steamed vegetables, mushrooms, tomatoes, and pasta in large bowl.

3 In container of blender or food processor, combine the dressing ingredients. Cover and process at low speed until smooth.

4 Add dressing to pasta and toss gently to coat. Chill at least 1 hour before serving.

Nutritional information per serving
150 calories
70% of calories from carbohydrate
17% of calories from protein

13% of calories from fat
2 grams of fat
4 grams of fiber

* If you are unable to tolerate broccoli, replace it with green beans or another vegetable that you can tolerate.
** Yogurt is usually well tolerated, even if you are lactose intolerant. If you do not tolerate yogurt, take 1 lactase enzyme tablet with this salad or replace the yogurt with the same amount of low-fat mayonnaise. Remember that the salad will be higher in fat with low-fat mayonnaise.
*** This small amount of Parmesan cheese should be tolerated except in the case of a severe lactose intolerance. You may omit the cheese if desired.

39

Side Dishes
Salads and Vegetables

Apple Salad

Applejack Acorn Squash

Asparagus Salad

Boiled Potatoes with Apples

Broiled Tomato Halves

Carrot Salad

Cucumber-Radish Salad

Dilly Carrots

Eggplant in Rich Tomato Sauce

Green Beans Italian Style

Green Salad

Grilled Zucchini

Lemony Potatoes

Potato Salad

Snow Pea Salad

Spinach Salad

Steamed Broccoli with Orange Sauce

Sweet Potato Casserole

Vegetable Kabob

Veggie Stir-Fry

Apple Salad
SERVES 4

4 celery stalks, diced
8 ounce can of sliced water
  chestnuts, drained
4 tart apples, sliced (either red or
  green are attractive)
2 tablespoons low-fat mayonnaise

*6–8 tablespoons plain nonfat or
  low-fat yogurt
1 teaspoon lemon juice
½ teaspoon ground cinnamon
¼ teaspoon ground ginger

1   Place celery, water chestnuts, and apples in medium-sized serving bowl.

2   In small bowl, mix together mayonnaise, yogurt, lemon juice, and spices. Pour over the apple mixture.

3   Chill and serve.

Nutritional information per serving

132 calories
78% of calories from carbohydrate
6% of calories from protein

16% of calories from fat
3 grams of fat
4 grams of fiber

Applejack Acorn Squash
SERVES 4

2 medium acorn squash
¼ cup applejack, apple brandy, or
  another apple flavored liqueur

2 tablespoons brown sugar
2 teaspoons butter or margarine

1   Preheat oven to 350°.

2   Cut squash in half and remove seeds. Place on baking sheet.

3   Mix applejack and brown sugar together. Spoon into center of each squash half, dividing the mixture evenly.

4   Put ½ teaspoon of butter in center of each squash.

5   Bake for 1 hour or until soft, basting occasionally.

Nutritional information per serving

157 calories
84% of calories from carbohydrate
5% of calories from protein

11% of calories from fat
2 grams of fat
4 grams of fiber

---

* Yogurt is usually well tolerated by lactose intolerant individuals. If you would prefer not to use the yogurt, you may replace with additional low-fat mayonnaise, but this will be higher in fat.

Asparagus Salad
SERVES 4

Although the percentage of fat in this salad appears high, the grams of fat are actually low because the total calories are so low.

1 pound asparagus, washed	2 teaspoons sesame oil
1½ tablespoons white rice vinegar	¼ teaspoon salt, if desired
1½ tablespoons dry vermouth	2 teaspoons white rice vinegar

1   Cut each asparagus spear in 3 to 4 pieces each. Cut on the diagonal, rolling the spear halfway around after each cut.

2   Heat vinegar (1½ tablespoons) and vermouth in medium skillet. Bring to a bare simmer. Add asparagus and sauté for about 2 to 3 minutes. Remove from heat.

3   Place asparagus into serving bowl. Add oil, salt, and additional vinegar. Toss and chill.

Nutritional information per serving

49 calories	41% of calories from fat
38% of calories from carbohydrate	3 grams of fat
21% of calories from protein	1 gram of fiber

Boiled Potatoes with Apples
SERVES 4

2 large baking potatoes, sliced ½ inch thick	½ teaspoon salt
1 medium onion, diced	2 tart apples, chopped (do not peel)
1 cup water	1 teaspoon cider vinegar

1   In medium saucepan simmer potatoes and onion in salted water for 10 minutes.

2   Add apples and cook for an additional 10 minutes.

3   Drain any remaining water and gently stir in vinegar. Serve.

Nutritional information per serving

160 calories	2% of calories from fat
91% of calories from carbohydrate	less than 1 gram of fat
7% of calories from protein	5 grams of fiber

Broiled Tomato Halves
SERVES 4

2 large tomatoes
4 tablespoons whole wheat
breadcrumbs

1 teaspoon oregano
2 teaspoons balsamic vinegar

1 Preheat broiler.
2 Cut tomatoes in half.
3 Mix together breadcrumbs, oregano, and vinegar. Divide evenly and spread over tomato halves.
4 Broil 4 inches from heat source for about 5 minutes or until top is browned.

Nutritional information per serving

38 calories
75% of calories from carbohydrate
14% of calories from protein

11% of calories from fat
less than 1 gram of fat
1 gram of fiber

Carrot Salad
SERVES 4

1 pound carrots, peeled and sliced
on diagonal
½ cup chopped parsley
3 tablespoons raspberry vinegar
4 teaspoons olive oil

2 teaspoons Dijon style mustard
1 teaspoon sugar
¼ teaspoon ground cinnamon
lettuce

1 Steam carrots until crisp-tender, about 5 to 7 minutes.
2 Toss carrots and parsley together in medium-sized serving bowl.
3 Whisk together remaining ingredients in small bowl. Pour over carrots and parsley.
4 Refrigerate for several hours before serving. Serve on a bed of curly lettuce.

Nutritional information per serving

97 calories
53% of calories from carbohydrate
6% of calories from protein

41% of calories from fat
5 grams of fat
4 grams of fiber

Cucumber-Radish Salad

SERVES 4

1 cucumber, peeled and deseeded
½ pound radishes
½ cup cilantro, chopped

4 tablespoons white rice vinegar
2 tablespoons mirin
½ tablespoon sesame seed oil

1   Slice cucumbers and radishes paper thin. Mix with chopped cilantro in a serving bowl.
2   Mix remaining ingredients together and pour over vegetables. Chill 1 to 2 hours in refrigerator before serving.

Nutritional information per serving

42 calories
56% of calories from carbohydrate
7% of calories from protein

37% of calories from fat
2 grams of fat
3 grams of fiber

Dilly Carrots

SERVES 4

6 medium carrots, scraped and
   sliced

½ cup grapefruit juice
¼ teaspoon dried dill

1   Steam carrots until almost tender, about 5 to 7 minutes.
2   Heat grapefruit juice to boiling in small skillet. Add carrots and cook at medium high heat until the juice is nearly evaporated, about 2 to 3 minutes.
3   Add dill, stir, and serve hot.

Nutritional information per serving

60 calories
88% of calories from carbohydrate
8% of calories from protein

4% of calories from fat
less than 1 gram of fat
4 grams of fiber

Eggplant in Rich Tomato Sauce

SERVES 4

If you hate to open a can of tomato paste when only 1 or 2 tablespoons are called for in a recipe, here's the solution: the remainder can be frozen in tablespoon portions in small plastic bags.

1 teaspoon olive oil

1 medium onion, chopped

1 medium eggplant, peeled and cut into 2 × ½ × ½-inch strips

1 medium green pepper, coarsely diced

2 tablespoons soy sauce

2 tablespoons tomato paste

1 tablespoon lemon juice

¾ cup water

1   Heat oil in saucepan and cook onion for 1 to 2 minutes over medium heat.

2   Add eggplant and green pepper and cook, stirring frequently, until eggplant is almost tender, about 10 minutes. Add water as necessary to prevent sticking.

3   Add remaining ingredients and stir until well mixed. Cover and cook until flavors are well blended and eggplant is soft, about 5 minutes. Serve.

Nutritional information per serving

58 calories

65% of calories from carbohydrate

14% of calories from protein

21% of calories from fat

2 grams of fat

3 grams of fiber

Green Beans Italian Style

SERVES 4

2 cups green beans, cut in 1-inch pieces

½ cup onion, chopped

1 cup chopped tomato

1 teaspoon oregano

½ cup chicken stock, preferably homemade (see page 208)

Put all ingredients in saucepan. Cook over medium heat until green beans are tender, about 10 minutes. Serve.

Nutritional information per serving

40 calories

70% of calories from carbohydrate

21% of calories from protein

9% of calories from fat

less than 1 gram of fat

2 grams of fiber

Green Salad

SERVES 4

You'll find this to be a very interesting and delicious salad. It is time-consuming but worth the effort!

4 small heads of Belgian endive, washed and torn into bite-sized pieces

1 cup sorrel, washed and stems removed, torn into bite-sized pieces

½ cup chopped fennel

10–12 basil leaves, chopped

1 tablespoon finely chopped lemon peel

4 teaspoons lemon juice

4 teaspoons sparkling water or club soda

4 teaspoons white vinegar

4 teaspoons olive oil

¾ cup fresh or unsweetened frozen, thawed, and well-drained blueberries

1   Mix endive, sorrel, fennel, basil, and lemon peel together in large salad bowl.

2   In medium bowl, whisk together lemon juice, water, vinegar, and oil. Add ½ cup of blueberries and mash with a spoon. Strain and discard pieces of blueberry.

3   Pour dressing over salad and garnish with remaining blueberries.

Nutritional information per serving

65 calories

33% of calories from carbohydrate

6% of calories from protein

61% of calories from fat

5 grams of fat

2 grams of fiber

Grilled Zucchini

SERVES 4

2 whole zucchini

2 teaspoons olive oil

1½ teaspoons oregano

½ teaspoon salt (if desired)

*¼ teaspoon black pepper

1   Cut zucchini into quarters lengthwise. You will have 8 long pieces of zucchini.

2   Mix together oil, oregano, salt, and pepper. Brush each zucchini section lightly.

3   Place on heated grill, pulp side down, and grill for 5 to 8 minutes or until soft but not mushy. Serve immediately.

Nutritional information per serving

36 calories

33% of calories from carbohydrate

13% of calories from protein

54% of calories from fat

2.4 grams of fat

2 grams of fiber

---

* Black pepper is a gastric irritant. Omit the pepper if you find it to be irritating, and use dried basil instead.

Lemony Potatoes
SERVES 4

12 small new potatoes, cleaned and unpeeled
½ cup defatted chicken stock, preferably homemade (see page 208)

*1 teaspoon grated lemon peel
1 tablespoon chopped fresh parsley
*¼ cup lemon juice
1 teaspoon cornstarch

1 Boil potatoes until tender.

2 In small saucepan, heat stock, lemon peel, and parsley.

3 Mix lemon juice with cornstarch until thoroughly blended. Add this to broth, stirring constantly over low heat until slightly thickened.

4 Place potatoes in serving dish and pour lemon sauce over top. Toss lightly to coat all potatoes.

Nutritional information per serving

125 calories
90% of calories from carbohydrate
9% of calories from protein

1% of calories from fat
less than 1 gram of fat
2 grams of fiber

Potato Salad
SERVES 4

1½ pounds small red-skinned potatoes
**½ cup 1% low-fat cottage cheese
***¼ cup plain nonfat or low-fat yogurt
½ teaspoon dried dill

2 teaspoons low-fat mayonnaise
1½ teaspoons Dijon style mustard
¼ cup chopped onion
¼ cup chopped fresh parsley
2 tablespoons minced green pepper (optional)

* Lemon may be irritating to the esophagus.
** If you are lactose intolerant, purchase low-lactose cottage cheese or take 1 lactase enzyme tablet with this meal.
*** Yogurt is usually well tolerated by lactose intolerant individuals. If you cannot tolerate yogurt, replace with an additional ¼ cup of low-fat mayonnaise. This will increase the recipe's fat content.

1   Steam unpeeled potatoes until fork tender. Do not overcook.

2   While potatoes are steaming, place the cottage cheese, yogurt, dill, mayonnaise, and mustard in the blender and blend until smooth.

3   Drain potatoes when cooked. Cut them into bite-sized pieces, taking care not to tear the skins.

4   Combine potatoes, onion, parsley, and green pepper in bowl. Pour dressing over top and toss lightly.

Nutritional information per serving
190 calories
78% of calories from carbohydrate
16% of calories from protein

6% of calories from fat
1 gram of fat
2 grams of fiber

Snow Pea Salad
SERVES 4

SALAD

½ pound snow peas, washed and strings removed

*½ pound (about 20) young corn spears, sliced on diagonal

¼ cup finely chopped fresh coriander (cilantro)

¼ cup finely chopped fresh parsley

DRESSING

1 teaspoon brown sugar
¼ cup rice wine vinegar

1 teaspoon soy sauce
1 tablespoon sesame oil

1   Mix peas, corn, coriander, and parsley together in medium-sized serving bowl.

2   Mix dressing ingredients together in small bowl. Pour over vegetables.

3   Refrigerate for at least 1 hour before serving.

Nutritional information per serving
109 calories
58% of calories from carbohydrate
11% of calories from protein

31% of calories from fat
4 grams of fat
4 grams of fiber

* Available in oriental food stores or the specialty food section of your grocery store. They are more digestible and cause less gas and discomfort than regular corn.

Spinach Salad

SERVES 4

Although this salad appears to be high in fat, it is actually much lower than a typical salad as the amount of oil is less than usual. The salad will be lower in fat if you omit the walnuts.

8 cups fresh spinach leaves,
    washed and torn
*1 grapefruit, sectioned,
    membranes removed
**¼ cup walnuts, chopped

1 tablespoon olive oil
1 tablespoon wine vinegar or
    balsamic vinegar
1 tablespoon lemon juice
1½ teaspoons honey

1   Place spinach in salad bowl. Arrange grapefruits and walnuts on the spinach.

2   In small bowl, whisk together oil, vinegar, lemon juice, and honey.

3   Pour dressing over salad. Toss and serve.

Nutritional information per serving

130 calories
35% of calories from carbohydrate
13% of calories from protein

52% of calories from fat
8 grams of fat
4 grams of fiber

Steamed Broccoli with Orange Sauce

SERVES 4

***1 pound broccoli, stalks peeled
    and sliced on diagonal, florets
    cut into bite-sized pieces
****½ cup orange juice
¼ cup dry white wine

½ medium onion, chopped
¼ teaspoon thyme
1 teaspoon cornstarch
1 teaspoon cold water

1   Steam broccoli until tender.

2   While broccoli is cooking, place orange juice, wine, onion, and thyme in saucepan and simmer until onion is translucent.

* Grapefruit may be irritating to the esophagus.
** Nuts are often gas producing. You may be able to tolerate this small amount, but the recipe will work equally well without the nuts.
*** Broccoli can be gas producing. You may substitute any other vegetable that you find easier to tolerate, such as green beans or carrots.
**** Orange juice may be irritating to the esophagus.

3   Mix cornstarch with cold water. Add cornstarch mixture to orange juice mixture. Cook until thickened, stirring constantly.

4   Place cooked broccoli spears in serving dish. Pour orange sauce over broccoli and serve.

Nutritional information per serving

50 calories

70% of calories from carbohydrate

24% of calories from protein

6% of calories from fat

less than 1 gram of fat

4 grams of fiber

Sweet Potato Casserole

SERVES 4

2 cups cooked, mashed sweet potatoes

1 cup crushed pineapple, drained

2 tablespoons brown sugar

*¼ teaspoon ground cloves

1   Preheat oven to 400°.

2   Stir together all ingredients.

3   Coat baking dish with nonstick vegetable oil spray and add sweet potato mixture.

4   Bake for 25 minutes and serve.

Nutritional information per serving

235 calories

93% of calories from carbohydrate

5% of calories from protein

2% of calories from fat

less than 1 gram of fat

3 grams of fiber

Vegetable Kabob

SERVES 5

KABOBS

20 cherry tomatoes

20 whole mushrooms

2 large green peppers, cut in 20 square pieces

* Cloves can be replaced with allspice.

Sauce

*¼ cup plain nonfat yogurt
**2 teaspoons tahini

1 teaspoon lemon juice
¼ teaspoon coriander

1 Arrange vegetables on skewer in the following order: tomato, mushroom, pepper, tomato, mushroom, pepper. Repeat to total 10 skewers.

2 Coat broiler pan with nonstick vegetable oil spray. Lay kabobs on pan.

3 Broil kabobs about 3 minutes per side.

4 While vegetables are broiling, mix sauce ingredients together, stirring until smooth.

5 Serve kabobs and sauce separately, allowing each person to drizzle sauce over vegetables as desired.

Nutritional information per serving (2 kabobs and 1 tablespoon sauce)

52 calories
55% of calories from carbohydrate
21% of calories from protein

24% of calories from fat
2 grams of fat
3 grams of fiber

Veggie Stir-Fry
SERVES 4

1 tablespoon olive oil
1 medium onion, thinly sliced
1 medium red potato, unpeeled,
    cut in half lengthwise, then
    thinly sliced crosswise

1½ cups mushrooms, sliced
½ teaspoon basil
4 cups spinach leaves, washed and
    well drained
soy sauce to taste

1 Heat oil in wok or large skillet. Cook onion and potato over medium high heat, stirring frequently. Add water to wok as needed to prevent sticking.

2 When potatoes are partially cooked, add mushrooms and basil. Continue stirring as vegetables cook.

3 When potatoes and mushrooms are almost cooked, add spinach and soy sauce. Cook until spinach is done and remove from heat. Serve.

---

* Yogurt is usually well tolerated by lactose intolerant individuals. If you are unable to tolerate yogurt, you could take 1 lactase enzyme tablet with the kabobs, or use a sauce of tahini, lemon juice, and coriander.
** Tahini is a sesame seed paste available in specialty food stores, Middle Eastern markets, and health food stores.

Nutritional information per serving

115 calories	30% of calories from fat
60% of calories from carbohydrate	4 grams of fat
10% of calories from protein	4 grams of fiber

40 Breads and Muffins

Banana Bran Bread

Blueberry Orange Bread

Easy Corn Bread

Oat Biscuits

Oatmeal Raisin Muffins

Pumpkin Muffins

Banana Bran Bread
YIELD: 16 SLICES

½ cup unprocessed wheat bran
*½ cup buttermilk
2 tablespoons softened margarine
½ cup sugar
1 whole egg
2 egg whites
2 medium ripe bananas, mashed

1½ teaspoons vanilla
½ cup unbleached white flour
½ cup whole wheat flour
1 tablespoon baking powder
½ teaspoon baking soda
½ teaspoon salt
½ teaspoon ginger

1 Preheat oven to 350°.
2 Prepare loaf pan by lightly greasing with margarine or coating with nonstick vegetable oil spray.
3 In small bowl, soak bran in buttermilk for 15 minutes.
4 In medium bowl, cream the margarine, sugar, and eggs. Add mashed banana, vanilla, and bran mixture and mix well.
5 In large bowl, sift together dry ingredients and spices. Add wet

---

* Buttermilk is usually well tolerated by lactose intolerant individuals because it is cultured. The total amount of buttermilk is also very small in this recipe.

ingredients to dry ingredients and mix until combined. Do not over-mix.

6   Pour into a 9 × 5 × 3-inch loaf pan and bake for 50 minutes.

Nutritional information per serving (1 slice)

92 calories	19% of calories from fat
71% of calories from carbohydrate	2 grams of fat
10% of calories from protein	2 grams of fiber

Blueberry Orange Bread

YIELD: 15 SLICES

If you are using frozen blueberries, it is important to drain them well. Start draining them several hours before you plan to make the bread.

2 tablespoons butter or margarine	1 cup unbleached white flour
¼ cup boiling water	1 cup whole wheat flour
½ cup orange juice	1 teaspoon baking powder
1 tablespoon finely chopped	¼ teaspoon baking soda
orange rind	½ teaspoon salt
1 egg	1 cup fresh or thawed, well-
1 cup sugar	drained, frozen blueberries

1   Preheat oven to 325°.
2   Melt butter in boiling water in small bowl. Add juice and rind.
3   In large bowl, beat egg with sugar until light and fluffy.
4   Sift flour, baking soda, baking powder, and salt together into small bowl.
5   Add dry ingredients alternately with orange liquid to the egg and sugar mixture. Mix blueberries in gently.
6   Bake in 9 × 5 × 3-inch loaf pan that has been coated with nonstick vegetable oil spray.
7   Bake for 1 hour and 10 minutes. Turn out onto rack to cool. Slice when completely cool.

Nutritional information per serving (1 slice)

133 calories	14% of calories from fat
79% of calories from carbohydrate	2 grams of fat
7% of calories from protein	2 grams of fiber

Easy Corn Bread

YIELD: 9 PIECES

1 cup yellow cornmeal	½ teaspoon salt
1 cup whole wheat flour	2 egg whites
¼ cup granulated sugar	3 tablespoons vegetable oil
1 tablespoon baking powder	*1 cup skim milk

1 Preheat oven to 400°.

2 Coat a 9-inch-square, 2½-inch-deep baking pan with nonstick vegetable oil spray.

3 In medium bowl, stir together the cornmeal, flour, sugar, baking powder and salt until well mixed.

4 In small bowl, beat together egg whites and oil until blended. Stir in the milk. Very gently, stir the egg-milk mixture into the dry ingredients until well blended but not overmixed. Spoon batter into prepared pan, smoothing and spreading the top out toward the edges.

5 Bake for 18 to 20 minutes, or until the bread is tinged with brown and is springy on top. Cut into pieces and serve while warm.

Nutritional information per serving (1 piece)

168 calories	27% of calories from fat
62% of calories from carbohydrate	5 grams of fat
11% of calories from protein	2 grams of fiber

Oat Biscuits

YIELD: 12 BISCUITS

This is significantly lower in fat than a typical biscuit.

1 cup unbleached white flour	¼ cup rolled oats
3 tablespoons sugar	⅓ cup oat bran
1 tablespoon baking powder	2 tablespoons margarine
½ teaspoon salt	*¾ cup skim milk

1 Preheat oven to 425°.

2 Coat a 9-inch-round baking pan with nonstick vegetable oil spray.

* Use lactose-reduced milk if you are lactose intolerant.

3 Sift flour, sugar, baking powder, and salt into a medium bowl. Add oats and oat bran. Cut in the margarine with two butter knives and blend until mixture is crumbly.

4 Make a well in the center of the flour mixture. Pour in the skim milk. Stir quickly, but gently, just until dough comes together. The dough should be moist but pliable.

5 Turn out the dough onto a lightly floured sheet of waxed paper. Fold the waxed paper over the dough and gently pat to a thickness of about ¾ inch.

6 Cut biscuits, using a floured 2-inch-round biscuit cutter or glass. Place on prepared pan.

7 Bake for 15 minutes or until golden brown. Serve immediately.

Nutritional information per serving (1 biscuit)

83 calories	23% of calories from fat
66% of calories from carbohydrate	2 grams of fat
11% of calories from protein	1 gram of fiber

Oatmeal Raisin Muffins

YIELD: 1 DOZEN

1 cup rolled oats	1¼ teaspoon baking powder
*¾ cup buttermilk	½ teaspoon baking soda
2 tablespoons softened margarine	½ teaspoon salt
2 egg whites	½ teaspoon cinnamon
⅓ cup brown sugar	**⅛ teaspoon ground nutmeg
⅓ cup orange juice concentrate	***1 cup seedless raisins
1 cup whole wheat flour	

1 Preheat oven to 400°.

2 Prepare muffin tins with paper liners or coat with nonstick vegetable oil spray.

3 In medium bowl, soak rolled oats in buttermilk for 15 minutes.

4 In medium bowl, cream margarine, egg whites, brown sugar, and orange juice concentrate. When thoroughly mixed, add to oat mixture.

5 In large bowl, mix dry ingredients and spices.

---

* Buttermilk is usually well tolerated by lactose intolerant individuals because it is cultured. If you are unable to tolerate buttermilk you can treat it with lactase enzyme drops 24 hours before making this recipe.

** Omit the nutmeg if you are unable to tolerate it.

*** Raisins can be gas producing. If you prefer to omit the raisins, increase the brown sugar to ½ cup.

6 Add wet ingredients and raisins to dry ingredients, mixing only enough to thoroughly combine. Do not overmix.

7 Bake for 15 to 20 minutes.

Nutritional information per serving (1 muffin)

155 calories	15% of calories from fat
75% of calories from carbohydrate	3 grams of fat
10% of calories from protein	3 grams of fiber

Pumpkin Muffins

YIELD:1 DOZEN

2 tablespoons margarine	1 cup unbleached white flour
½ cup brown sugar	2 teaspoons baking powder
1 egg	½ teaspoon baking soda
1 egg white	1 teaspoon cinnamon
*1 cup buttermilk	¼ teaspoon ground ginger
½ cup canned pumpkin	**¼ teaspoon ground nutmeg
1 cup whole wheat flour	**⅛ teaspoon ground cloves

1 Preheat oven to 400°.

2 Prepare muffin tins with paper liners or coat with nonstick vegetable oil spray.

3 In medium bowl, cream margarine, brown sugar, egg, and egg white. Add buttermilk and pumpkin and mix well.

4 In large bowl, combine dry ingredients and spices. Mix well to ensure adequate distribution of the leavening agents and spices.

5 Add wet ingredients to dry ingredients. Mix until combined, but do not overmix.

6 Fill muffin tins three-quarters full and bake for about 25 minutes.

Nutritional information per serving (1 muffin)

144 calories	17% of calories from fat
72% of calories from carbohydrate	3 grams of fat
11% of calories from protein	2 grams of fiber

---

* Buttermilk is usually well tolerated by lactose intolerant individuals because it is cultured. If you are unable to tolerate buttermilk you can treat it with lactase enzyme drops 24 hours before making these muffins.

** These spices can be eliminated from recipe if they are irritating for you.

41 *Breakfast Dishes*

Berry Banana Smoothie

Brown Rice Cereal

Buttermilk Wheat Pancakes

Frosted Melon Cooler

Fruit Cup

Granola

Hot Buckwheat Cereal

Lemon Pancakes

Orangy French Toast

Strawberry Pancakes

Tomato, Mushroom, and Basil Omelet

Berry Banana Smoothie
SERVES 1

*½ cup plain nonfat yogurt
**½ cup skim milk
1 small ripe banana, cut in chunks
⅓ cup strawberries, cut in half
   (blueberries or raspberries
   would also work well)

1 teaspoon maple syrup
3 ice cubes

* Yogurt is usually well tolerated by lactose intolerant individuals. If you cannot tolerate yogurt, take 1 lactase enzyme tablet with this drink.
** Use low-lactose milk if you are lactose intolerant.

Combine all ingredients in blender and process until smooth and thick. Serve.

Nutritional information per serving

245 calories

77% of calories from carbohydrate

19% of calories from protein

4% of calories from fat

1 gram of fat

4 grams of fiber

Brown Rice Cereal

SERVES 4

This is a great way to use up leftover rice, especially on a cold winter morning.

4 cups cooked brown rice

2 tablespoons maple syrup

*1 cup skim milk

2 peaches, sliced, or 1 cup canned peaches in their own juice

1 Combine all ingredients in medium saucepan.

2 Bring to a boil, turn heat to medium, and cook to desired thickness, about 8 minutes. Serve warm.

Nutritional information per serving

302 calories

86% of calories from carbohydrate

10% of calories from protein

4% of calories from fat

1 gram of fat

7 grams of fiber

Buttermilk Wheat Pancakes

SERVES 4

⅔ cup unbleached white flour

1⅓ cups whole wheat flour

1 teaspoon baking powder

½ teaspoon baking soda

½ teaspoon salt

**2 cups buttermilk (or a little more, if needed)

4 teaspoons vegetable oil

1 Stir dry ingredients together in a medium bowl until thoroughly mixed.

* Use low-lactose milk if you are lactose intolerant.

** Buttermilk is usually well tolerated by lactose intolerant individuals because it is cultured. If you are unable to tolerate buttermilk you can treat it with lactase enzyme drops 24 hours before making these pancakes.

2 Beat the buttermilk and oil together until blended. Gently stir buttermilk mixture into dry ingredients until thoroughly blended but not overmixed. If the batter seems too thick, thin it with a bit more buttermilk until a pourable but still fairly thick consistency is achieved.

3 Lightly oil and preheat a griddle. Pour batter onto hot griddle and cook until bubbles form on the top surface and the bottoms are browned (about 60 to 70 seconds). Turn over with a spatula and cook about 1½ more minutes or until cooked through and nicely browned. Serve warm with maple syrup or fruit.

Nutritional information per serving
300 calories
66% of calories from carbohydrate
15% of calories from protein

19% of calories from fat
6 grams of fat
6 grams of fiber

Frosted Melon Cooler

SERVES 1

1 cup cantaloupe, fresh or frozen
  (thawed)
1 cup ice

¼ cup apple juice concentrate
¼ cup water

Combine all ingredients in blender and whip until frothy. Serve.

Nutritional information per serving
168 calories
92% of calories from carbohydrate
4 % of calories from protein

4% of calories from fat
less than 1 gram of fat
2 grams of fiber

Fruit Cup

SERVES 6

1 medium apple, cored and diced (peeled if desired)
1 medium pear or peach, cored, pitted, and diced
1 banana, peeled and sliced
*10 ounce can of mandarin oranges, drained
**½ cup seedless grapes (halved if desired)

½ cup blueberries, fresh or frozen
¼ cup frozen lemonade concentrate (any other juice concentrate would also be acceptable)
***¾ cup plain low-fat or nonfat yogurt

1 Prepare fruits and place in a large bowl. (The fiber content will be higher if the skins are left on the fruit.)
2 Mix lemonade concentrate with yogurt. Pour over fruit and toss lightly.

Nutritional information per serving

110 calories
87% of calories from carbohydrate
7% of calories from protein

6% of calories from fat
1 gram of fat
3 grams of fiber

Granola

YIELD: 5 CUPS

Granola is traditionally high in fat because it usually has more oil or margarine than this recipe, as well as nuts and coconut.

2 tablespoons margarine
2 tablespoons water
¼ cup honey
1 teaspoon cinnamon

3 cups rolled oats
1 cup grapenuts
****½ cup raisins

* Oranges may be irritating to the esophagus; omit if you are unable to tolerate them.
** Grapes are a gas producing fruit. You may want to substitute ½ cup of melon for the grapes.
*** Yogurt is often well tolerated by lactose intolerant individuals. If you are unable to tolerate yogurt, take 1 lactase enzyme tablet with this salad.
**** Raisins are gas producing. If you are unable to tolerate raisins, use chopped dried apples or apricots instead.

1 Preheat oven to 350°. While oven is preheating, melt margarine in 9 × 13-inch baking pan. Remove from oven.

2 Stir water, honey, and cinnamon into margarine until well blended.

3 Stir oats and grapenuts into margarine mixture until grains are well coated.

4 Bake for 15 minutes until oats are lightly browned. Stir twice during baking time to prevent uneven browning.

5 Remove from oven and stir in raisins. Cool. Serve with nonfat or lactose-reduced milk or with fruit juice.

Nutritional information per serving (½ cup)

202 calories	17% of calories from fat
73% of calories from carbohydrate	4 grams of fat
10% of calories from protein	3 grams of fiber

Hot Buckwheat Cereal
SERVES 2

This is a wonderful, hearty breakfast for those mornings when you need a lot of energy. It's great before a day of skiing.

5 cups water	1½ teaspoons minced orange peel
1 cup whole buckwheat (kasha)	1½ teaspoons ground cinnamon
2 apples, unpeeled, diced	

1 Bring water to boil in 3-quart saucepan. Add buckwheat, stirring, and return to boil. Reduce heat to medium and cook uncovered for about 8 minutes, stirring occasionally.

2 Stir in diced apples, orange peel, and cinnamon. Continue to cook about 3 to 5 more minutes or until most of the liquid has evaporated.

3 Serve topped with skimmed milk or low-lactose skimmed milk. (If you would prefer not to use any milk at all, only cook the buckwheat an additional 2 to 3 minutes after adding the apples. It will then be a thinner consistency.)

Nutritional information per serving

260 calories	6% of calories from fat
85% of calories from carbohydrate	2 grams of fat
9% of calories from protein	8 grams of fiber

Lemon Pancakes

YIELD: 18 PANCAKES

PANCAKES

1 cup unbleached white flour
1 cup whole wheat flour
2½ tablespoons sugar
1½ tablespoons baking powder
½ teaspoon salt
¼ cup unprocessed wheat bran

2 egg yolks
*2½ cups skim milk
2 tablespoons melted margarine
grated rind of 1 lemon
2 egg whites, stiffly beaten

1 In large bowl, sift flour, sugar, baking powder, and salt. Add bran and mix.
2 In medium bowl, beat egg yolks until creamy and stir in milk, margarine, and lemon rind.
3 Stir egg yolk mixture into flour mixture using as few strokes as possible.
4 Fold in egg whites thoroughly.
5 Drop batter onto hot griddle coated with nonstick vegetable oil spray. Bake until bubbly on surface. Turn and brown on the other side.
6 Serve with lemon-honey topping.

LEMON-HONEY TOPPING**

YIELD: 2 CUPS

1 tablespoon cornstarch
¾ cup water
¼ cup lemon juice

1 cup honey
***dash nutmeg

1 Whisk cornstarch into water and lemon juice.
2 Heat until thickened, stirring constantly.
3 Add honey and nutmeg. Stir.
4 Serve hot over pancakes.

Nutritional information per serving (3 pancakes, 3 tablespoons topping)
376 calories
74% of calories from carbohydrate
11% of calories from protein
15% of calories from fat
6 grams of fat
4 grams of fiber

* If you are lactose intolerant, use lactose-reduced milk
** This topping should not be used by individuals with esophageal irritation.
*** Nutmeg can be replaced with cinnamon.

Orangy French Toast *

SERVES 6

TOPPING

1 cup mandarin oranges in light
    syrup

¾ cup maple syrup

FRENCH TOAST BATTER

2 whole eggs
2 egg whites
2 cups orange juice
**1½ cups skim milk
¼ cup sugar

½ teaspoon vanilla
1 tablespoon Grand Marnier
1 pound loaf of day-old French
    bread cut into 1½-inch diagonal
    slices

1   Place topping ingredients in saucepan and let simmer over low heat.

2   Separate eggs and beat whites (4) until thick but not stiff.

3   Whisk egg yolks, juice, milk, sugar, vanilla, and Grand Marnier together. Fold in the thickened whites.

4   Cut bread. Add bread to the egg mixture and let soak for 10 minutes on each side.

5   Coat medium skillet with nonstick vegetable oil spray. Heat over medium heat. Add bread slices to skillet and cook on each side until golden brown.

6   Serve topped with orange syrup.

Nutritional information per serving
    478 calories
    80% of calories from carbohydrate
    11% of calories from protein

9% of calories from fat
5 grams of fat
2 grams of fiber

* Individuals with esophageal irritation should not make this recipe.
** If you are lactose intolerant, use lactose-reduced milk.

Strawberry Pancakes
SERVES 4

1 egg or 2 egg whites
*1¼ cups buttermilk
1 tablespoon melted butter or
  margarine
¾ cup whole wheat flour, sifted
½ cup unbleached white flour,
  sifted

¼ cup unprocessed wheat bran
1 teaspoon sugar
2 teaspoons baking powder
½ teaspoon baking soda
½ teaspoon salt
1 cup sliced strawberries, frozen or
  fresh

1   In large bowl, beat egg with electric mixer at high speed.
2   Add buttermilk and margarine or butter and beat for 1 minute.
3   Add remaining ingredients except berries and mix by hand, until just blended.
4   Add berries and mix.
5   Cook on hot griddle using ¼ cup batter for each pancake. You may have to coat griddle with nonstick vegetable oil spray.
6   Top pancakes with your favorite syrup, honeyed yogurt, or cottage cheese.

Nutritional information per serving (3 pancakes)

235 calories
65% of calories from carbohydrate
14% of calories from protein

21% of calories from fat
5 grams of fat
2 grams of fiber

Tomato, Mushroom, and Basil Omelet
SERVES 2

2 teaspoons olive oil
½ medium onion, chopped
½ cup chopped fresh mushrooms
1 small tomato, diced
1½ tablespoon chopped fresh basil
  or ½ teaspoon dried

2 egg yolks
4 egg whites
1 tablespoon seltzer water
fresh chopped parsley

1   Coat a nonstick skillet with a nonstick vegetable oil spray. Add the olive oil and heat. Sauté the onion until soft. Add the mushrooms,

---

* Buttermilk is usually well tolerated by lactose intolerant individuals because it is cultured. If you cannot tolerate buttermilk, or if you are severely lactose intolerant then add lactase enzyme drops to the milk 24 hours before making this recipe.

tomato, and basil and cook another 1 to 2 minutes. Remove from the heat.

2 Beat the egg yolks and egg whites with seltzer water.

3 Coat another nonstick skillet with nonstick vegetable oil spray and heat. Add eggs. Cook, stirring a few times and swirling the pan so that it is evenly coated with eggs, until the eggs are almost completely cooked.

4 Top the egg with the vegetable mixture. Tilt the pan to a 45-degree angle from the burner and using a fork push one edge of the omelet so that it rolls over the filling and into an oval shape. Continue cooking over low heat for about 1 minute. Tilt the pan so that the omelet rolls onto a serving plate.

5 Serve immediately, garnished with chopped parsley.

Nutritional information per serving

165 calories	56% of calories from fat
18% of calories from carbohydrate	10 grams of fat
26% of calories from protein	2 grams of fiber

42   *Desserts*

Apple Cake

Apricot Apples

Banana Dream Pie

Banana-Rhubarb Compote

Blueberry-Apple Crumble

Carrot Brownies

Chocolate Angel Cake

Oatmeal Drop Cookies

Patriotic Pizzazz

Peanut Butter Bars

Refrigerator Chip Cookies

Apple Cake
SERVES 8 TO 9

1 tablespoon softened margarine
¾ cup brown sugar
*¼ cup skim milk
1 egg
1 cup unsweetened applesauce
¼ cup unprocessed wheat bran
¾ cup unbleached white flour

¾ cup whole wheat flour
1½ teaspoon baking powder
¼ teaspoon baking soda
1½ teaspoon cinnamon
1 medium apple, peeled, cored, and chopped
¼ cup confectioners sugar

* Use low-lactose milk if you are lactose intolerant.

1   Preheat oven to 350°.

2   Coat 8 × 8-inch baking pan with nonstick vegetable oil spray.

3   In small bowl, cream together margarine and brown sugar. Add milk, egg, and applesauce. Mix well.

4   In large bowl, combine dry ingredients and cinnamon and mix well to ensure even distribution of the leavening agents.

5   Add wet ingredients to dry ingredients. Mix. Add apple and mix just until distributed.

6   Pour batter into pan and bake for 50 minutes or until firm.

7   Sift confectioners sugar over top after cake is completely cooled.

Nutritional information per serving

200 calories

83% of calories from carbohydrate

7% of calories from protein

10% of calories from fat

2 grams of fat

3 grams of fiber

Apricot Apples
SERVES 6

6 medium Granny Smith apples, washed, peeled, and cored

1 cup firmly packed light brown sugar

¾ cup apricot jam

3 tablespoons apricot brandy

*¼ cup slivered almonds

1   Preheat oven to 375°.

2   Place apples in 9 × 13-inch glass baking dish.

3   In small bowl, combine sugar and jam.

4   Place 1 to 2 tablespoons of sugar mixture in the center of each apple, filling halfway (you will have some left over).

5   Add ½ inch of water to baking dish.

6   Bake apples 20 minutes, basting with cooking liquid occasionally.

7   Add brandy to the remaining sugar mixture. Brush apples with sugar and brandy mixture.

8   Continue baking the apples about 20 minutes more or until soft.

9   Top apples with almonds and bake for 2 more minutes or until almonds are toasted.

* Nuts are often gas producing. You may be able to tolerate this small amount as a garnish however.

10 Transfer apples to plates. Pour cooking liquid into small heavy saucepan and boil to thicken, if necessary. Pour sauce over apples. Serve warm or at room temperature.

Nutritional information per serving

350 calories	7% of calories from fat
92% of calories from carbohydrate	3 grams of fat
1% of calories from protein	3 grams of fiber

Banana Dream Pie

YIELD: ONE 8-INCH PIE (SERVES 8)

CRUST

1½ cups graham cracker crumbs
½ cup All Bran cereal
½ cup orange juice

1 tablespoon melted margarine or butter

FILLING

*1 cup skim milk
1 envelope unflavored gelatin
**¾ cup part skim ricotta cheese

2 teaspoons vanilla
3 medium-sized *ripe* bananas
¼ cup sugar

GARNISH

2 kiwi fruit, peeled and sliced

8–10 fresh strawberries, sliced

1 Blend crust ingredients. Press crust over bottom and sides of 8-inch pie pan. Bake in 350° oven for 10 minutes. Cool.

2 Place ½ cup cold skim milk in small saucepan. Sprinkle gelatin on top. Let soak for 5 minutes. Heat and stir until gelatin dissolves.

3 In food processor or blender, combine gelatin/milk mixture with remaining ½ cup milk and other filling ingredients. Blend until smooth and creamy.

4 Pour into crust and chill for 1 hour. Remove and garnish with sliced kiwi and strawberries. *Note:* The top of the banana cream will discolor slightly from exposure to the air so the pie will have a better appearance if the garnish covers the entire top. Other garnish alternatives are fresh raspberries or low-fat yogurt.

5 Return to refrigerator to set for another 3 hours.

---

* Use lactose-reduced milk if you are lactose intolerant.
** If you are mildly lactose intolerant, you should tolerate the amount of ricotta cheese in one serving. However, if you are severely lactose intolerant, take 1 lactase enzyme tablet with this pie.

Nutritional information per serving

226 calories

69% of calories from carbohydrate

12% of calories from protein

19% of calories from fat

5 grams of fat

4 grams of fiber

Banana-Rhubarb Compote

SERVES 4

2 cups frozen rhubarb

*⅓ cup orange juice

⅓ cup honey

2 medium-sized bananas, sliced

**½ cup vanilla low-fat yogurt

***4 teaspoons minced walnuts

1 In medium saucepan combine rhubarb, orange juice, and honey. Cover and cook for 10 minutes.

2 Add sliced bananas, cover, and heat until bananas are warmed and softened.

3 Serve in individual dessert dishes with 2 tablespoons of vanilla yogurt on top, sprinkled with 1 teaspoon of finely chopped walnuts.

Nutritional information per serving

320 calories

90% of calories from carbohydrate

4% of calories from protein

6% of calories from fat

2 grams of fat

4 grams of fiber

Blueberry-Apple Crumble

SERVES 6

FILLING

2 tablespoons granulated sugar

1 tablespoon whole wheat flour

¼ teaspoon ground cinnamon

2 cups fresh or frozen blueberries
(thaw before using)

1 large tart apple, skin on, finely
chopped

---

* The small amount of orange juice shouldn't present a problem for individuals with esophogeal irritation.

** Yogurt is usually well tolerated by lactose intolerant individuals. If you cannot tolerate yogurt or prefer not to use it, sprinkle a small amount of powdered sugar on top as a garnish.

*** Most people find nuts to be gas producing. You may be able to tolerate a small amount as a garnish. If not, omit them.

Topping

⅓ cup whole wheat flour	1½ tablespoons vegetable oil
⅔ cup rolled oats	1–2 tablespoons water or apple
½ cup packed brown sugar	juice (if necessary)

1 Preheat oven to 375°.

2 To prepare the filling, stir together the granulated sugar, flour, and cinnamon in a 1½-quart baking dish. Stir in the blueberries and chopped apple until they are coated with the flour-sugar mixture. Set aside.

3 To prepare the topping, stir together the flour, oats, and brown sugar in a small bowl until well mixed. Stir in the oil until thoroughly incorporated. Mixture should clump together slightly so use the additional water or juice as necessary. Sprinkle the topping over the blueberry mixture.

4 Bake the crumble, uncovered, for 25 to 30 minutes or until bubbly at the edges and cooked through. Serve warm or at room temperature.

Nutritional information per serving

217 calories	17% of calories from fat
78% of calories from carbohydrate	4 grams of fat
5% of calories from protein	4 grams of fiber

Carrot Brownies

Yield: 24 squares

1 cup brown sugar	½ cup rolled oats
2 tablespoons margarine	½ teaspoon baking powder
1 egg	½ teaspoon baking soda
2 egg whites	2 cups finely grated carrots
1 teaspoon vanilla	1 cup confectioners sugar
*½ cup orange juice	**skim milk
1½ cups unbleached white flour	

1 Preheat oven to 350°.

2 Coat a 9 × 13-inch baking pan with nonstick vegetable oil spray.

* The small amount of orange juice shouldn't present a problem for individuals with esophageal irritation.
** Use low-lactose milk if you are lactose intolerant, although you will use such a small amount that it should not have any effect.

3 Mix sugar and margarine together in large bowl.

4 Add eggs, vanilla, and orange juice; beat.

5 Stir in dry ingredients and mix well. Stir in carrots.

6 Spread mixture into baking pan. Bake 30 to 35 minutes or until firm when pressed.

7 Place confectioners sugar in small bowl and add just enough skim milk to thicken. Drizzle over brownies while still warm.

Nutritional information per serving (1 square)

106 calories

82% of calories from carbohydrate

7% of calories from protein

11% of calories from fat

1 gram of fat

1 gram of fiber

Chocolate Angel Cake

SERVES 10

1 cup sifted flour

1 cup sugar

¼ cup cocoa, unsweetened

½ teaspoon salt

1½ cups egg whites

(approximately 6 medium)

1 teaspoon cream of tartar

1 teaspoon vanilla

confectioners sugar

1 Preheat oven to 325°.

2 Sift flour, sugar, cocoa, and salt *ten* times into a medium bowl. This step is essential to the success of the recipe.

3 With electric mixer, beat egg whites until frothy, add cream of tartar, and beat again by hand.

4 Fold in dry ingredients, and add vanilla.

5 Turn into an ungreased 10 × 4-inch tube pan.

6 Bake for about 1 hour and 15 minutes or until cake springs back when lightly touched. Invert pan for about 1 hour. Remove from pan and cook on rack.

7 If desired, sift confectioners sugar over top before serving.

Nutritional information per serving

130 calories

86% of calories from carbohydrate

11% of calories from protein

3% of calories from fat

less than 1 gram of fat

less than 1 gram of fiber

Oatmeal Drop Cookies

YIELD: 3 DOZEN

1 cup unbleached white flour
½ cup sugar
½ teaspoon baking powder
¼ teaspoon baking soda
½ teaspoon salt
½ teaspoon cinnamon
1 cup oats, regular or quick
  cooking

½ cup oat bran
*½ cup raisins
¼ cup vegetable oil
1 whole egg
2 egg whites
**⅓ cup skim milk
***¼ cup chopped walnuts

1 Preheat oven to 400°.
2 Sift flour, sugar, baking powder, baking soda, salt, and cinnamon together. Add oats and oat bran. Mix. Add raisins and mix.
3 In small bowl, beat oil, eggs, and milk until blended. Add wet ingredients to dry ingredients and mix until thoroughly blended.
4 Add walnuts, and stir.
5 Drop by heaping teaspoonful onto ungreased baking sheet about 1½ inches apart.
6 Bake 10 to 12 minutes.

Nutritional information per serving (2 cookies)
  129 calories
  57% of calories from carbohydrate
  10% of calories from protein
  33% of calories from fat
  5 grams of fat
  2 grams of fiber

Patriotic Pizzazz****

SERVES 4

This is a very elegant dessert, suitable for company.

* Raisins can be gas producing. You may want to substitute diced, peeled apples. Dice apples in ¼-inch cubes and reduce the milk to ¼ cup.
** Use low-lactose milk if you are lactose intolerant.
*** Nuts can be gas producing. They may be tolerated in these small amounts, but can be omitted if desired.
**** Individuals with esophageal irritation should not make this recipe.

1 pint strawberries
¼ cup confectioners sugar
2 cups lemonade

2½ cups blueberries
*¼ cup vanilla low-fat yogurt
fresh mint

1 Wash and hull strawberries, drain thoroughly, and cut into small pieces.

2 Put strawberries and sugar in a food processor or blender and puree until smooth.

3 Add enough lemonade to the strawberry puree to make 2 cups of liquid. Pour liquid into a plastic freezer container, cover, and put in the freezer. When the mixture begins to freeze around the sides of the container, after about 20 minutes, remove from the freezer and scrape the frozen bits into the center of the container to break up ice crystals. Return to freezer and freeze until firm but not solid, about 45 minutes.

4 While strawberry ice is setting, wash blueberries, drain thoroughly, place in food processor or blender, and puree. Strain and discard any seeds or skins.

TO ASSEMBLE DESSERT:

1 Pour about ⅓ of blueberry puree onto each of 4 chilled dessert plates, forming an even pool.

2 Place yogurt into a pastry bag with a round tip.

3 Pipe about a tablespoon dollop of yogurt in the center of the puree. Draw a toothpick through the yogurt at regular intervals, alternating from the edge of the puree to the center and then from the center of the dish to the edge, creating a web design.

4 Place 3 small scoops of the strawberry ice on the outside of the puree. Garnish with a fresh sprig of mint placed in the center of each scoop of ice.

5 Repeat to make 4 servings. Serve immediately.

Nutritional information per serving
167 calories
88% of calories from carbohydrate
8% of calories from protein

4% of calories from fat
less than 1 gram of fat
4 grams of fiber

* Yogurt is usually well tolerated by lactose intolerant individuals. If you are unable to tolerate yogurt, take 1 lactase enzyme tablet with this dessert.

Peanut Butter Bars

YIELD: 12 BARS, 2¼ × 2½ INCHES EACH

½ cup peanut butter
½ cup honey
2 tablespoons water
1 egg yolk
2 egg whites
½ teaspoon vanilla extract
½ cup unbleached white flour

½ cup dry rolled oats
½ cup grapenuts cereal (not flakes)
1 teaspoon cinnamon
2 teaspoons baking powder
¼ teaspoon baking soda
*½ cup seedless raisins

1 Preheat oven to 350°.
2 Coat 8 × 8-inch baking pan with nonstick vegetable oil spray.
3 In medium-sized bowl, beat peanut butter, honey, water, egg yolk, egg whites, and vanilla until smooth.
4 In large bowl, combine flour, oats, grapenuts, cinnamon, baking powder, and baking soda.
5 Add wet ingredients to dry ingredients and beat until combined.
6 Add raisins and stir to combine. Pour into baking pan and bake for about 20 minutes or until set.

Nutritional information per serving (one bar)
182 calories
59% of calories from carbohydrate
12% of calories from protein
29% of calories from fat
6 grams of fat
2 grams of fiber

Refrigerator Chip Cookies

YIELD: 3 DOZEN

Although these cookies are not low in calories, they have less than half the fat of a typical cookie and more fiber.

2 eggs
1 cup brown sugar, firmly packed
3 tablespoons vegetable oil
½ teaspoon vanilla
¾ cup unbleached white flour

1 cup whole wheat flour
¾ teaspoon baking powder
¼ cup mini chocolate chip
   morsels, semisweet

* Raisins may be omitted if you find them to be gas producing.

1   Beat eggs. Add brown sugar, oil, and vanilla. Beat.

2   Sift flour and baking powder into large bowl.

3   Add wet ingredients to dry and mix well (texture will be crumbly). Add chips and mix.

4   Shape with hands into a 2-inch-round roll. Wrap in waxed paper and refrigerate until firm.

5   Preheat oven to 375°.

6   Remove roll from refrigerator when firm and slice thin, into approximately 36 slices.

7   Bake on ungreased cookie sheet for 5 to 8 minutes or until golden brown.

Nutritional information per serving (2 cookies)

128 calories	26% of calories from fat
67% of calories from carbohydrate	4 grams of fat
7% of calories from protein	1 gram of fiber

43 Miscellaneous

Basic Vinaigrette Dressing

Cooked Salad Dressing

Marinara Sauce

Mock Sour Cream

Basic Vinaigrette Dressing
YIELD: 1 CUP

This very basic, easy to prepare dressing is something you will always want to keep on hand. When refrigerated, it will stay good indefinitely and tastes much better than bottled salad dressings. Use this on your tossed salads, grain based salads, and for basting or marinating your meats or poultry. The typical proportion of oil to vinegar in a salad dressing is 3 parts oil to 1 part vinegar. In order to keep the fat content lower, this proportion has been altered. If you have difficulty getting accustomed to more vinegar and less oil, start with a 1 to 1 ratio and make the change gradually. Use any type of oil or vinegar to change the flavor of this recipe, but always use the best quality!

10 tablespoons balsamic vinegar	pinch of basil
6 tablespoons extra virgin olive oil	pinch of thyme
4 teaspoons Dijon style mustard	*1 garlic clove, whole
½ teaspoon dried tarragon	

Whisk ingredients together and store in covered jar in refrigerator. Garlic should be left whole to flavor the dressing. Remove the garlic before serving.

---

* Garlic can be gas producing. If you are unable to tolerate it, the dressing is good even without the garlic.

Nutritional information per serving (2 tablespoons)

92 calories	94% of calories from fat
6% of calories from carbohydrate	10 grams of fat
0% of calories from protein	0 grams of fiber

Cooked Salad Dressing

YIELD: 1¼ CUPS

1 tablespoon cornstarch	1 cup cold water
1 teaspoon sugar	¼ cup catsup
*1 small garlic clove, finely chopped	3 tablespoons red wine vinegar

1   Combine cornstarch, sugar, garlic, and water in small saucepan and blend until cornstarch dissolves. Add catsup and vinegar.

2   Stir over medium heat at a slow boil until thickened. If you are not using garlic, add your herb(s) at this point and cook another minute. Remove from heat, place in small bowl, and refrigerate.

Nutritional information per serving (2 tablespoons)

10 calories	0% of calories from fat
100% of calories from carbohydrate	0 grams of fat
	0 grams of fiber
0% of calories from protein	

Marinara Sauce**

YIELD: 3½ CUPS STRAINED, 4 CUPS UNSTRAINED

1 tablespoon olive oil	6 ounces tomato paste
¼ cup chopped onion	4 ounces water
¼ cup chopped celery	2 tablespoons fresh parsley
*1 garlic clove, finely minced	1 tablespoon dried basil
3 cups whole canned tomatoes	1 teaspoon sugar

1   Heat oil in large saucepan. Sauté onion, celery, and garlic until softened.

---

* Garlic can be gas producing. If you are unable to tolerate the garlic, replace it with 1 teaspoon of one or more dried herbs of your choice, such as basil, dill, oregano, or tarragon.

** Individuals with esophageal irritation should not make this recipe.

2 Place remaining ingredients in food processor or blender and puree until smooth.

3 Add tomato ingredients to saucepan, cover, and simmer over very low heat for 45 minutes to 1 hour.

4 Serve the sauce as it is or, if you prefer, strain it to remove the seeds.

Note: If you have fresh basil on hand, omit the dried basil and add 3 basil leaves just before you cover to simmer.

Nutritional information per serving (½ cup)

58 calories	29% of calories from fat
59% of calories from carbohydrate	2 grams of fat
12% of calories from protein	1 gram of fiber

Mock Sour Cream

YIELD: ABOUT 1¼ CUPS

*1 cup 1% low-fat cottage cheese	1 tablespoon lemon juice
*2 tablespoons skim milk	

1 Combine all ingredients in blender. With blender on high speed, blend the mixture until smooth, about 2 minutes.

2 Chill in refrigerator for several hours before serving.

Nutritional information per serving (2 tablespoons)

18 calories	13% of calories from fat
20% of calories from carbohydrate	less than 1 gram of fat
67% of calories from protein	0 gram of fiber

Note: The same amount of regular sour cream has 62 calories and 6 grams of fat (87% of the calories are from fat).

* Use lactose-reduced products if you are lactose intolerant.

General Index

Page numbers in italics indicate illustrations on that page.

Weight *(cont.)*
  diet(s), 128, 171–74, 177
  fiber and, 124, 125

gain, 183–85
loss, unexplained, 25, 183–85

Yellow skin color, 24

Recipe Index

Acorn squash, applejack, 249
Acorn squash soup, 207–8
Angel cake, chocolate, 280
Appetizers, 207–12
Applejack acorn squash, 249
Apple(s)
  apricot, 276–77
  blueberry-, crumble, 278–79
  boiled potatoes with, 250
  cake, 275–76
  salad, 249
Apricot apples, 276–77
  Asparagus salad, 250

Banana
  berry, smoothie, 266–67
  bran bread, 261–62
  dream pie, 277–78
  -rhubarb compote, 278
Barley delight, 241–42
Barley salad, cold, 243
Basic chicken stock, 208–9
Basic vinaigrette dressing, 285–86
Beautiful bow tie pasta, 242
Beef
  kabobs, 221–22
  marinated and grilled flank steak, 223
  stew with cranberries, 222–23
  stir-fry orange, 223–24
  very veggie meatloaf, 225–26
Bell peppers, stuffed, 229
Berry banana smoothie, 266–67
Biscuits, oat, 263–64
Blueberry-apple crumble, 278–79
Blueberry orange bread, 262
Boiled potatoes with apples, 250
Bow tie pasta, beautiful, 242

Bran bread, banana, 261–62
Bread
  banana bran, 261–62
  blueberry orange, 262
  easy corn, 263
Breakfast dishes, 266–74
Broccoli, steamed, with orange sauce, 257–58
Broiled tomato halves, 251
Brownies, carrot, 279–80
Brown rice cereal, 267
Bulgur wheat salad, cold, 244
Buttermilk wheat pancakes, 267–68

Cake, apple, 275–76
Cake, chocolate angel, 280
Carrot(s)
  brownies, 279–80
  dilly, 252
  salad, 251
Cereal
  brown rice, 267
  granola, 269–70
  hot buckwheat, 270
Chicken
  breast, marinated and grilled, 239
  breasts in creamy mustard sauce, 232–33
  fajitas, 233–34
  and herbs baked in foil, 231–32
  lemonade, 238
  with mushrooms and sun-dried tomatoes, 235–36
  oriental barbecued, 239–40
  salad, fruited, 237
  stock, basic, 208–9
  -vegetable stir-fry, 234–35